THE
*f*ACELIFT*d*IARIES

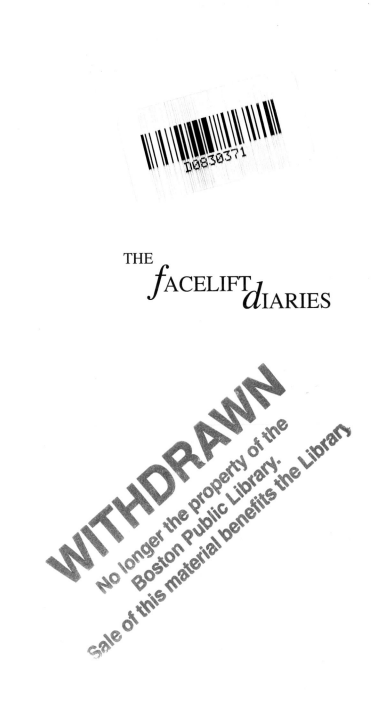

THE *f*ACELIFT *d*IARIES

WHAT IT'S *REALLY* LIKE TO HAVE A FACELIFT

JILL SCHARFF AND JAEDENE LEVY

BookSurge, LLC North Charleston, SC
Library of Congress Control Number: 2004104348

Designed by Jeff Schwaner.
Cover Design by Nancy D'Arrigo.

To order additional copies, please contact us.
BookSurge LLC
www.booksurge.com
1-866-308-6235
orders@booksurge.com

For all the WWHHPS
and all who are wondering...

ACKNOWLEDGEMENTS

Our heartfelt thanks go to our surgeons Jorge Reisin and John William Little for taking great care of our faces and giving each of us what we want. We are also grateful to Elaine, Kit, Pat, Randye, and Rosie, for assisting them in helping us get a good result and for holding our hands when we couldn't see. In the diaries, we've used other names for them and some of our friends so as not to be too specific, but we want to give them full credit here. Our husbands, Chuck and David, and our children Daniel, Kate, Nell, Marjorie, Stephanie, Xanthe, and Zoe totally came through for us, and we love them for it and for everything else. Thanks to all our friends, especially Meg Cooper, Shelley Doctors, Brent Goo, Barbara Rein, and Judy Simmons for their active support, and to Eddy Brez, Shelley Levi, and Kate and Nell Scharff for their enthusiasm and notes on early drafts. Stephanie Levy and Zoe Scharff gave us written responses from which we have borrowed gladly. Linda Cashdan, Jan Clarkson, Stan Corwin, Kim Kanner, and Homer Moyer who know all about books encouraged us when we needed it most. Last but not least, we are grateful to Anna Innes who smoothed our manuscript's submission, and to Jeff Schwaner and Nancy D'Arrigo who gave our text its facelift.

CONTENTS

Before the Facelift

The Facelift Diaries

After the Facelift

*b*EFORE THE *f*ACELIFT

1

Who We Are

WE'RE HAVING A FACELIFT, AND WRITING ABOUT IT FOR YOU, whoever you are, wherever you are in your thinking about YOUR face. We're going to tell you how we found our plastic surgeons, how we talked to our families, and how we helped each other through it all. We want to share the story of our surgeries and our healing, our fears, hopes, and satisfactions, and the camaraderie of doing it together. Whether you make the same decision we made or not, you will think about it, because, whenever a facelift is mentioned, people get right into it.

We're therapists, and we know how women feel and what they don't tell their friends or their doctors. We're also patients — we know how we feel and we know our doctors don't tell us everything. Our journey covers the surgical details of course, but we also deal with the overlooked emotional and social aspects. For something often considered superficial, a facelift conversation brings us to a surprisingly more intimate level with other women. Once a woman knows you've had a facelift, she feels connected to you. Once she knows, she claims the right to examine your face openly and make comments. A facelift puts you out there, and asks you to look into yourself.

You may be a woman like us, over fifty, who finds that the look of your face doesn't match how you feel about yourself. Unlike us, you may not need or want a facelift, or you may be scared to have it. You may be opposed to it, unable to make time for it, or unable to convince your partner that it's worth the risk and the expense. You may worry about how others will view you if you choose to have a facelift or decide not to. You may be a young woman for whom the prospect is far off. You may want to have a facelift and not know who to ask about it. Whoever you are, wherever you stand, we're inviting you to join us on this journey.

The unvarnished truth

Women normally don't tell all about their facelifts, and neither do their surgeons. The advertisements you read in magazines typically include photos of "before" (awful) and "after" (awesome) — and nothing to show for the six months in between. We're not going to make plastic surgery seem like a miracle, because we aren't selling the idea. We simply want to tell you what it is REALLY like. We give you the unvarnished truth.

It isn't an easy process. We don't gloss over that fact. It isn't pretty. "Scabs are gross," one of our daughters says, and we agree with her, but they are part of life, and we think it's helpful to be honest. We complain about suffering sometimes, but it feels good to be able to complain and have a friend to complain to. The healing process doesn't go along smoothly.

It goes up and down and back and forth. We'll tell you about worries, some suffering, family strain, moments of depression and self-doubt, tears and laughter. We'll give a much more real view than you would ever get from a doctor. You might as well know all about it ahead of time.

What is a facelift?

The full facelift consists of a brow lift, upper and lower eyelid lifts, the facelift, the necklift, body fat insertion to fill out the hollows, and laser. A partial facelift (also called a mini-lift) comprises one or some of these components. Many women do their eyes only, maybe in their forties or younger, some choose a brow lift with their eye lift, and a few do only the lower part of their face, or only the neck. Doctors don't want to do only the neck because you might look at yourself later and see that your face is too old for your neck.

Who wants to go through multiple surgeries and anesthetics? We don't, but maybe you do. If you like the idea of incremental boosts, then that's for you. You may think you're saving time and money that way, but you won't in the long run, because doing it in dribs and drabs is time-consuming and expensive. We believe in doing the whole thing at once, especially if you want to do it only once.

A word of caution

There are some terrible facelifts. There are some doctors who don't do such a good job. It's awful to imagine you might turn out like that. You've got to make it your business to talk to a number of people and look at them and find out the names of their doctors. Making sure your surgeon is Board Certified is a safety measure, but it's better to know

who did what to whom. We think that the worst results are
due to multiple procedures, but that's not what we're talking
about. This book is not for the facelift veteran. This is for the
facelift beginner.

To the restored face

The facelift experience touches every aspect of life. You
can hardly imagine how all-encompassing it is. Some of you
might say that it is better not to know, or you might never
venture it. We say "No"; you feel more scared by what you
don't know. Our friends who read this book appreciate our
candor; our daughters don't. They say they will never have
it done. Of course they say that; they don't need it. Young
women may not yet empathize with women of our genera-
tion because they don't yet know what women experience.
They want to distance themselves from the facelift procedure and from the kinds of pain and trauma older women go
through for beauty. Women put up with a lot without necessarily thinking of it as suffering. Think of the happy ending:
A restored beautiful face.

It's two months for Jaedene, and six months for Jill,
before we feel comfortable in our faces. Until then, healing is
hard work, physically and emotionally, and we benefit from
having each other to talk to about it. We let you in on that
conversation. We are aware that there are many women in
this country who want to know about this but don't have
someone to talk to about it. What we say to you is, "Come
on and we'll tell you all about it." WE will be your compan-
ions.

We touch on many facets of our experience. You don't
have to be our age to join us. You can come in and sample
the experience of being together, talking like this about our

concerns. We will tell you what it is like to be a woman facing this decision, and how we get through the process of healing with one another and with our family and friends. Ours is a voyage of personal discovery, a journey in friendship that we want to share with you.

Body and soul

In our professional lives as psychotherapists we believe in looking inside ourselves and learning from experience. We believe that talking about fears, longings, and conflicts is helpful in reaching peace and mastery. So we reflect on how we feel and why, and we talk to each other about it. If the inner life is so important to us, then why are we having face-lifts? It's obvious. How we feel is reflected in how we look. And our looks no longer match the way we feel. How we look and feel about ourselves affects how much enjoyment we can have.

We don't need to be therapists to know that physical beauty is only skin deep. Who you are inside is the most important thing in life and love. But we don't believe it's the only thing that matters. We also love good make-up, stylish clothes, perfume, great shoes, and hair color. To us, our appearance is part of who we are. We want to please ourselves and appeal to others. We want our inner and outer selves to match. Over fifty, it gets harder to feel that. Our inner vitality isn't shining through our wrinkled skin. Time for a face-lift.

With children already gone from the house and both of us working, we are in a financial position to pay our facelift bills. Other healthy people want a facelift, but think they can't afford it. Not necessarily true, now that monthly payment plans make the $119 a month facelift as accessible as orthodontics. We have the health to do it. For us, it's a choice, and one that we want to make. We are glad we are able to do as we please.

Our concern for each other deepened nine years ago when we helped each other recover from surgery the same month. We commiserated on the telephone, encouraged each other, and finally celebrated our recoveries. That's how we became close. That time, we were seriously ill and we had to have surgery to save our lives. That time it was an emergency.

This time it's a choice. Elective plastic surgery is different than emergency surgery. First of all you have time to think about it. Secondly you don't desperately need it, so choosing to put your life at risk is a big responsibility.

Feeling apprehensive

Of course we feel apprehensive. We ask a million questions. What are we doing? What will our husbands think? What if, what if....? We worry that recovery from plastic surgery will be as painful as from our previous surgeries and anesthetics that we required to keep us alive. So what if we have scars from that? We are still here! But doing the Face is a choice we make simply to look better, and we are afraid that we may cause trouble for ourselves. "If anything happens to me, I'll never forgive myself!" If you get a nasty scar after a tummy tuck, you can hide it from people. With a facelift, you don't know ahead of time how it will turn out, and you can't hide the way you look. Not only that, you have to look at what you've done to yourself every day. We're facing our fears fair and square, and now it's time to get on with it.

Surgery has dealt well with our life-threatening illness, and so surgery can surely deal with our faces. We aren't afraid of the knife: it helped us before. We aren't afraid of pain:

though we both hate Demerol. We know what it is to feel weak during recovery. A facelift is surely a breeze compared to emergency surgery. We can do this.

So here we are again, helping each other prepare for and recover from surgery. It's still a big deal, but this time it's a lot different, because it's our choice. That time surgery was about not dying. This time it's about living.

*j*ILL
Our facelift sleuthing

For the past two years, Jaedene has been noticing which of her friends in Washington and New York had "work done." She loves to astonish me by pointing out the results of various procedures among acquaintances. I tease her about being "sophisticated and in-the-know." She teases me by calling me "brilliant but socially naïve." It's something of a game between us. She impresses and entertains me with her state-of-the-art knowledge, and I feel privileged to be brought into the fold, but I think Jaedene is gossiping. One day I realize that she is interested in a facelift for herself. She wants to join in but she is scared, but I don't yet know why. Unlike Jaedene, I am not frightened to have a facelift, but I have no idea how to go about it.

One day I ask Jaedene to sit down and talk seriously. A month later, our first facelift conversation finally takes place.

Coming straight to the point, Jaedene asks, "What is it you don't like about your face, Jill?"

"My frown. You should see me on videotape. I look really awful. Tired, old, disapproving, irritated. Put the video on pause and you can count the wrinkles on my forehead — all 14 of them! And they aren't shadows from the lighting, like I wish. When I look in the mirror they are all still there.

"I said to my husband, 'Look at these wrinkles. They really are the way they look on the video.' Guess what David said to me: 'That's not half so bad as the way your neck and chin look. Maybe it's time for a facelift.' Ouch!"

Jaedene is sympathetic but quickly warms to his point of view. "Go for it. Your husband supports it! My husband thinks it's crazy. Chuck can't see anything wrong."

Neither do I. Jaedene looks positively glamorous to me. "What would you like to have done to your face?" I ask.

"I don't like the wrinkle at the side of my mouth and the fold underneath my chin. And my eyes look tired all the time.

"I'm going to find out who people are going to."

Coming to terms with the choice

It is another month before we begin to have our first appointments, a month for me to realize that my husband is right and the time is now. It takes three months for Jaedene to choose her surgeon and reassure her husband, and six more months before we find the time in which to have the surgery. That gives us plenty of time for thinking it over and facing our fears. We want to look more attractive, but we don't want to become objects of scrutiny. We don't relish having to deal with envy if the facelift goes well, or pity if it doesn't. We don't want to need a facelift, but the truth is that we do, and so we have to find out more about it.

We don't want to be superficial in our choices or expectations of what surgery has to offer us. We want to be certain that we're making the right decision. Are we victims, trapped in our class and culture? Are we trapped in the Venus complex, blindly subscribing to the modern American beauty myth, trying to look like everyone else? Do we feel compelled to look a certain way? NO! We don't expect perfection. We just want to look better. We aren't looking for a magical change, we already enjoy our work and our families, and we lead meaningful lives. Having a facelift will be a way of living more visibly again and having the power of choice over our options.

We know that it involves much more than fixing the face on the outside. It's also about the "me" that's on the inside. It's about how we react and cope under stress. It's about our relationships with family and friends, the work we do with our patients or clients, our hopes for what lies ahead, and our fears about the future.

Here's our map of the territory for you.

2

Why We Want Our Facelifts

jILL
My father, my aunt

i TAKE AFTER THE SAVEGE FAMILY. DAD'S DEEP WRINKLES DIDN'T BOTHER HIM. He used to joke about planting potatoes in his furrowed brow. With spreading nostrils and falling cheeks, he had a face like a bulldog, which was quite grand in its way, but not one I would want! The aging Savege face that he felt fine about did not sit well on Auntie Dorrie, either. It's unfair that society holds men and women to different standards of beauty as they age. I used to think that I would never give in to that. But as I'm getting older, I find that the jowls that emphasized my father's masculinity do not enhance my femininity at all.

Now I know what Auntie Dorrie felt! She hated her dewlaps and wattles. But she lived in Edinburgh and she didn't know anyone who had had a facelift, or where to go to get one. Auntie Dorrie didn't need a facelift to improve her life any more than I did, but if she had lived in the United States, she would have had one, I'm sure.

When I went to arrange her funeral last year, I saw her in her coffin. Her skin was drawn tight over her cheekbones and her chin. In death she had had her facelift. I vowed that I wouldn't wait that long.

JAEDENE
My mother, myself

I am looking at a black and white photograph of my mother in her thirties. She is with the actress Rita Hayworth on the evening before her wedding to the Aly Khan, and my young mother holds her own. Rita is gazing up at my mother; my mother is looking at the camera. They are very beautiful women. How many people could join in with those two? As I look at this picture, I cannot imagine anyone competing with her in the beauty department.

I was always tremendously proud of her, but there was no way I could compete. So, I took myself out of the contest, without ever having gotten into it, and competed in other ways — verbally and scholastically. People were always saying to me, "Do you know what a beautiful woman your mother is?" Of course I did! It gave her access to social situations like the one in the photograph. It was how she used her beauty. Growing up, I heard these comments made about my mother and I saw how other women behaved with her. There was admiration and flattery, but there was cruelty too. And I realized that my mother was confused and hurt by the reactions to her. It was safer where I was, not particularly beautiful, but pretty enough to be noticed. I enjoyed that. It made me feel good about myself. It's not a question of being desperate for adulation. We all need that kind of feedback for self-esteem.

Now I am no longer being looked at by men, or women. And I miss that. As I grow older I am more appreciated for my intellectual abilities. I like that, and it makes me feel better than ever about myself, but I want the outside to match the inside. So, why not try to recapture my appearance? As I become more aware of the power I now have, I want back the power I once had. I can pay for it. So why not have a facelift? But, once again, there is fear. If I look better, will some women envy me? Giving myself the right to make the choice, will I seem too powerful? Or, worse yet, less feminine?

I want my face improved, but I don't want to give up anything for it. I only want to add things to my life, unless I choose to forfeit them. But there really isn't any safe place "in the middle."

*J*AEDENE
Visible and connected

In my family tradition, connecting with others socially is expected and prized. Friends are important to me. I usually enjoy being with people I know and meeting people I don't know. Yes, I'm very connected to the people I care about, and already know. But I feel less visible in settings with people I do not yet know, and may wish to get to know. And, if I become even less visible, it will be harder to connect. It will require a greater effort. A facelift might give me higher visibility and ease my way. But if I am too visible, people (women in particular) may disconnect, feeling that I have separated myself from them by having the surgery. So if I want a facelift, I want not too much of one. I want to find a place where I can stay safely ensconced somewhere "in the middle."

Jill
Staying in the game

I'm happy that David is supportive, but does that mean he is too interested in my improvement? Am I doing this to keep his attention? I don't think so, because although he's interested in looks, he also cares about intelligence, competence, and physical and mental fitness. So how am I doing in those areas?

I can still think clearly and creatively and I can still dance until the music stops, but I can't lift a 50-pound bag of mulch any more, and my memory isn't what it used to be. So I challenge my muscles to keep up by lifting weights and I stimulate my brain by learning Spanish. A new face won't cure my "senior moments." It won't turn back the clock. And it won't make me happy unless I'm happy anyway. But my face is something I can fix. Fixing it gives me power over one aspect of my being.

I'd rather earn respect through talent and hard work than get favors because of my looks. On the other hand, I don't like it that some patients think I am judging them harshly because of my frown, when I am simply concentrating and trying to see things from their point of view. I don't want my looks to detract from my image of competence. And I want that competent image to be definitely female. I don't want a crumpled face that says I'm old and makes me feel less feminine than I am.

Not that I'm looking for beauty or glamour. What I want is style and substance. The tailored classic approach suits me. What I want is to have my face neatened up. I don't want a memorable face. I want a feminine face. I want a face that looks okay, that I can take for granted. I want back the face I can forget about.

My only worry is, what if I lose the face I remember? What if I never look like myself again? What will that do to my identity?

JAEDENE
The invisible woman of a certain age

I was always a facelift "cheerleader," jumping up and down encouraging my friends to go for it, glad that I didn't need it. One day I realized that I could no longer look into the mirror and see my whole face.

Now I can only see what needs fixing — the puffs under my eyes, the deepening lines at the sides of my mouth, and the "crevices" radiating from my lips. I look into the mirror and squint so the puffs diminish. My hands automatically pull the sides of my face back and up. That's when I decide that I need to get into the ring. It's time to be a contender.

I have lots of mixed feelings about it. Does wanting to have my face "done" turn me into "a woman of a certain age?" Does thinking about it mean that I am already there? Neither appeals to me, because being a woman of a certain age is not something to aspire to in our society. It means not really being SEEN any longer, and in some cases, not being heard either. But I've already had conversations with my husband and friends about those issues. My husband can't imagine my not being seen or heard (though sometimes HE doesn't see or hear me), and my girlfriends know exactly what I'm talking about, because they have had those feelings too, and they hate them.

What if I have a facelift? Will I look into the mirror and see the kind of face I recognize too easily — the face that has clearly been "done", as indicated by the too-smooth, pulled look, with hair always combed forward to cover the scars? The kind of face that I gossip about?

Does wanting a facelift mean that I am a superficial person, someone without deep thoughts and mature under-standing, someone lacking in acceptance of nature and life's realities? I don't think so. Surely I can enjoy my maturity — but fight back for a little while longer.

3

What Our Loved Ones Feel

JILL
How dare you? It's the American Way!

*N*OW IN THEIR LATE TEENS AND TWENTIES, OUR YOUNGER CHILDREN, the ones who still come home during the summer, have complex reactions to the news of my facelift. They think the idea is gross, but they accept my choice. Then when I tell them I've booked a date in early summer — a time that's easiest on my patients who are often away on vacation anyway — the reality hits them. Zoe argues that this time will be a major cause of suffering for kids who have to live at home while doing internships this summer. Xanthe, who'll be away until fall, says she is sorry she won't be there to help me. Daniel says, "Don't expect me to be sorry for you. Put it this way. Let's say I'm sitting here eating my cereal and all of a sudden I decide to just SMASH my face down onto the counter and into the bowl, would you feel sympathy for me? No, because I had done it to myself. So that's why I think it's dumb. Do what you want, and I'll still speak to you, but don't expect sympathy from me."

My Scottish mother always said my grandmother had smooth skin until her death at 87, and I say that my mother, who is active at 87, has skin like that too. I'm never sure if she does or if it's a family myth passed on by one doting daughter to another. Anyway, Mum sees no need for a facelift. And even if she did, it's not in the Scottish repertoire. She says, "What on earth do you want to do a thing like that for? You don't need that. You look so young to me." I say, "Mum, it's the American way." She says, "Well I won't tell anyone. That's the Scottish way."

Mum had minor face surgery herself. It was for a precancerous growth. Now her eyesight is failing and she's waiting to have laser treatment for her retina without any guarantee of success. I admire her spirit, but I feel badly for her compared to me. We each have our concerns of aging, but mine are less serious than hers, and I can get the treatment I want without waiting.

Mum says I don't really need a facelift. I want to believe her. Maybe I don't need it yet. It isn't until Yolanda — an attractive Latin American psychotherapist, ten years younger than I am, shows up with a reconstructed face that I begin to think that sooner would be better. I'm not the only one who notices the improvement in Yolanda and its implications for me. When Kate, my step-daughter whose face isn't 40 yet, meets Yolanda, she turns to me and says, "You really need a facelift, Jill."

David agrees. Both his parents had successful face surgery. His father had to have an eyelid lift. His mother had her eyes and face done when she was my age. She is in full support of my doing the same. She is also encouraging David to accept his opthalmologist's referral to a plastic surgeon for an opinion about his eyes. Not that David is following up on it. One rule for him, one rule for me. Okay, it's enough for one of us to think about cosmetic surgery.

My friend Meg feels scared for me. She touches her own face in sympathy as if it is being cut. Catherine, who is on weekly chemotherapy says, "I wish I could do it too, but I'm not sure whether a person who's living with breast cancer can do something like that." Shelley says, "I envy your courage." Judy says, "How exciting!" Yolanda tells me what it was like for her.

I tell Jaedene, "Yolanda says, 'Oh yes, you should do it. You will be happy. I had no pain, just tightness. It was funny. I looked like E. T. with two maids taking care of me, putting cucumbers on my eyelids and crushing pineapples for me to drink. You will love it.' She made it sound like a party where she was queen for a day. It won't be like that here, but I think I'm going to do it."

Jaedene says, "Me too! We'll talk."

(We did talk, and that's what led to this book).

*j*AEDENE
You're crazy, you could die

When I first tell my mother I am planning to have a facelift, she says that I have a lot of courage. She tells me she thought about having it done years ago, but didn't have the nerve because after plastic surgery her friend went into a coma for years, and then died. By the end of the conversation my mother is telling me she loves me even if I'm a jerk for taking the chance.

My husband, Chuck, thinks I'm crazy to fight nature. But mostly, he is scared. Scared that I might start looking more closely at other men. Scared that I will die during all those hours of anesthesia. He keeps telling me to wait until next year. "What for?" I ask. He hopes I will somehow change my mind.

My daughters think it's crazy too. Stephanie tells me I'm beautiful, and I shouldn't change anything. Marjorie says, "Why would you do that? You're already married, Daddy thinks you're hot, and anyway, he's too old to see!"

Wasn't I pretty enough? No, that's not it. It's that something bad might happen to me. They are all thinking of the problem I had with the anesthetic five years ago... and no one has figured out why that happened.

In short they don't see the need for change. They are too worried about losing me.

4

Face-to-Face with Our Surgeons

*j*AEDENE
Shopping around

i START ASKING AROUND. I ASK MY FRIENDS ABOUT THEIR SURGERY. Who did it? What was it like? Have they gotten the results they hoped for? Anything they would change? I speak to friends who have friends who've had a facelift. What have they heard? How do their friends look? Do they all look the same? Some women tell me about a "friend" if they don't want to admit that they themselves had it done.

Jill and I have many facelift conversations. I talk and she listens. I report on doctors and the faces they have done. She goes to the first person whose name I give her, and that is it. One-stop shopping for her. Not me. I shop around. Many people think the best plastic surgery is in Texas, but that's too far away for me. Others go to New York where some doctors are doing a shorter operation, and I could easily go there. In the end, I have consultations with three plastic surgeons, all board certified in plastic surgery, articulate, specific about their "method", and attractive, having had some plastic surgery done on themselves. I pay close attention to see if they are listening to me. I like them all.

The choice of a plastic surgeon is a highly personal thing and not necessarily a reflection on the surgeon's skill and qualifications. For instance, my friend Ruth from New Jersey comes with me to see the surgeon in New York, and she likes him too, but in the end she decides she's more comfortable with another surgeon. It's a matter of personal fit, convenience, and confidence.

Finally, I decide. I want to be at home to recuperate, so the doctor has to be in my city. I have to see that other faces my surgeon has done don't look pulled. I have to understand what he will do and how he will do it. He and I have to agree on what needs to be done. I have to feel sure that he has heard me. And I think of one more thing. Will he be willing to work alongside an orthopedic surgeon so I can get rid of a ganglion on my wrist at the same time? I choose Dr. A in Bethesda, close to home.

Let me decide

I tell Dr. A I just want to look refreshed. He confirms that I look tired because my eyebrows are low and that vertical wrinkling at the center of my forehead is giving me an angry, worried look. The surgeon in New York said I didn't need a brow-lift. Dr. A says that the most important thing is to give me a brow-lift. He would do that by making the incisions for it in three places above my forehead. They would be short, starting near the hairline and going from front to back. I agree to that.

Then he mentions that I need a facelift and a neck-lift as well. The other incisions for these procedures would be behind my ears, in front of my ears, and along the hairline at the sides of my neck. I agree to that. Now Dr. A talks about cheek implants to counteract a hollow look that develops under the eyes with aging, but I don't want puffy cheeks. In that case, he would add a little fat from my abdomen to cheeks and brows instead. He wants to laser under my eyes, and above my upper lip to smooth out the small wrinkles. Before surgery I will have two appointments with his skin specialist who will vacuum my face. I am skeptical but it is supposed to make a difference.

I tell Dr. A over and over again that I want him to be conservative with my face, that when he's finished, I want to complain that he hasn't done enough. He says that there would then be nothing to complain about! We compromise. He agrees to no artificial cheek implants. I agree to a brow-lift, a little added fat to the cheeks, a facelift, neck-lift, and laser.

As for how I feel about his fee — my face is more important than a new car.

*j*ILL
One stop shopping

Jaedene puts me in touch with Marie whose face looks amazingly young, and natural. I never suspected she had a facelift. Marie highly recommends Dr. B, the downtown surgeon whose name Jaedene gave me. "He's passionate about his work, and he's a perfectionist, a bit of a fanatic. As far as my face was concerned, a fanatic was fine by me." He sounds fine for me too.

Dr. B is about my age and has a ponytail. His manner, however, is professorial, not Hollywood. First I make sure he is certified by the American Board of Plastic Surgery. I see from his bio that he publishes, teaches, and volunteers for surgical missions to developing countries. I like that.

He holds a mirror to my face and asks what I am worried about. Smiling sheepishly, I show him the drooping eyebrows and lids, the forehead frown and furrows, and the jowls. He explains that the smile is a natural facelift, and so he asks to look at my face without its smile. The more he looks and I comment, the more problems I notice — bags under the eyes, sagging cheeks, falling nose, and crumpled chin and neck. I like the way he addresses each concern, and then tells me about his surgical technique and how it would apply in my case. I'm a physician, and so I need all the details.

Like good surgeons today, Dr. B wants to avoid a startled or unnatural look. That's why he prefers not to do a central forehead lift with a long incision across the top of the face. In fact, he keeps most of the forehead wrinkles because they are expressive. He does a lateral brow-lift (at the sides of the forehead) using two small slits, one above each temple, running side-to-side behind and parallel to the hairline. He tightens the forehead by attaching it to two small screws above the temples. (Yes, screws!) If he needs to reduce the frown between the eyebrows, he adds a third small slit just behind the widow's peak at the front and center of the scalp, and reaches down from there to clean out the frown area.

When he lifts the neck and chin area, he makes an incision below the chin and another behind each ear, coming

33

around the lobe of the ear, and ending below the sideburn, a hidden incision that allows for any hairdo, even upswept styles.

Working on the cheeks, he makes four incisions inside the mouth to reach up to the fat and muscle below the eyes. He tightens the muscles and moves fat back into its natural position and fixes it to peeled-back tissues over the bones of the face. (This is the part of deep technique that makes for a longer recovery process, I now know). By supporting the skin on fat and muscle, he avoids drawing the facial skin tightly to the skull.

He takes a graft from behind the ear to fill the hollow left after removing the bags of fat below the eyes. He recycles all the fat for use in the restoration of the face. He doesn't like to use implants. He takes some fat from the hip and grafts it under the lips and chin to fill in those lines that lipstick leaks into. Lastly he uses laser under the eyes and around the mouth and chin — not the forehead where he says it will not help. He will go light on the laser because my blue eyes tell him my skin is sensitive.

Dr. B's method seems better than simply pulling the skin taut, fastening it down, and cutting off the excess, as if the only problem is that the old skin is now too large for the face and could be corrected by trimming it like a pie-crust. The pie-lid won't sit well if the fruit inside sinks. I like his volumetric approach that conserves the natural curve and contour of the face. I choose Dr. B.

Three kinds of facelifts

I've learned that there are three types of facelift. The Skin-lift tightens the skin, trims off the excess, and holds the skin on the stretch with tension stitches. When it sags, the facelift

Questions to ask your surgeon

- *Describe what you will do and how you will do it*
- *Will you do all my surgery yourself?*
- *Will I have a mini-, skin-deep, or deep-tissue lift?*
- *Do you plan to use implants?*
- *Will you be taking away fat or adding fat?*
- *Will you use laser?*
- *Will you use screws temporarily or permanently?*
- *How much improvement can I expect realistically?*
- *How long will I be on the table?*
- *What is your fee?*
- *What does the operating room cost?*
- *What is the anesthesiologist's fee?*
- *Will my health plan pay for any of this? (Probably not)*
- *Can you recommend a good nurse?*
- *How do I reach you after office hours?*
- *Who covers for you?*
- *When will I be recognizable?*
- *Will there be emotional and psychological reactions?*
- *Is this it, or will there be corrections after the surgery?*
- *Is there anything else I haven't asked about?*

needs to be repeated. The SMAS lift combines work on the skin with work on the strong tissue that lies deep to the skin and above the muscle, tightening it to support the skin and the fat. The Deep-plane lift combines the skin lift and the SMAS lift with the technique of peeling back the tissues that cover the cheekbones, lifting them up, and folding them back on themselves, reattaching to them the muscles and fat in their new location. Your surgeon may use a few traditional incisions along a continuous line or multiple short ones.

Keep my face the way it is but change it

I tell Dr. B, "I see why you feel I need added fat to fill out my wrinkled cheeks, but I liked the slimness in my lower cheeks where the baby fat fell away by the time I was 40. The 30 year-old face with the choochie-cheeks is not the one I want to aim at."

Dr. B has never heard of choochie-cheeks, but he knows what I mean. He prefers a sculpted look too.

"How long would I be under anesthesia?" I ask.

"Maybe six hours, maybe nine. You may have heard of some surgeons who take two or three hours, but that's for a surface lift. I take as long as I need to get the best possible result."

"Do you think I could go back to work at four weeks?"

"You may feel well enough to work even at two weeks, and the bruising will be minimal at three weeks, but you'll look red, and swollen, your lips will be out to here, and don't be surprised if you don't look like yourself. One side may heal at a different rate than the other and you may feel-lopsided for a while. This could be disconcerting to your patients. Your recovery will take longer than for a mini-lift or a surface lift. I work with the deeper tissues, and they take time to heal."

That makes sense. I'm used to waiting patiently and I have good pain tolerance. I can do this.

"You're looking at about five weeks until you'll feel comfortable seeing patients," he continued, "but it'll be eight weeks at least before your family feels you are back to being you, and four months before the face settles, and really it's a year for complete healing."

I don't take in anything after "at least," and I fix my sights firmly on eight weeks.

His receptionist chimes in, "When I had mine done, I came back here at two weeks, all bruised and swollen, but hey, I fit right in here!"

But an unrecognizable face wouldn't fit in at my office at all. In my work as an analyst, I see my patients two to four times a week, and many of them look at me quite intently. I wouldn't want to freak anyone out.

"I suppose you wouldn't want to tell your patients about your procedure. Analysts don't answer questions, do they?" Dr. B continued.

> **What We Hope the New Face Will Say and Do**
>
> *A better-looking face can't cure depression*
> *But it changes how you join in relationships and work,*
> *Changes the responses to you.*
>
> *Choosing a facelift is a way of facing reality,*
> *Taking charge of your appearance,*
> *Staying in the social game,*
> *Competing in the professional world.*
>
> *A better looking face says to the world, "Look again, I'm here, I count, I'm to be reckoned with."*

He's right. I wouldn't like questions directed to me. I like to stay in the background, as neutral a presence as possible. I want to focus on the patient and on the inner person, not on externals, and certainly not on me. I don't want my concerns to intrude. I don't want to be selfish and vain.

The question I have to face is this: "You are a psychoanalyst who works on changing the inside. What on earth are you doing wanting a facelift?" True, I deal with the inner world of feelings and conflicts. I'm committed to the in-depth, slow process of self-healing that analysis or intensive psychotherapy offer. I'm totally against a quick fix for suffering, like using medication without psychotherapy. But I don't think face surgery is a quick fix for aging. I'll still be working on my physical, mental, and emotional fitness with exercise, reading, and self-analysis. It's just that I want my face to look the way I feel.

First of all I have to come to terms with admitting to myself that I want to make this choice and why, before I can think about whether to tell my patients. I won't be able to disguise the changes, so how can my facelift be a secret? I will have to tell my patients I am having elective face surgery to interrupt some of the signs of aging typical of my family. I want to spare them and me the worst of the visuals, and so I will take a couple of months off to give my face time to look more like myself.

I realize that I have decided. This is the 25th anniversary year of my practice. I will give myself not only a facelift, but also a mini-sabbatical — a time for reflection, attention to body and mind through study, writing, and travel in preparation for the next 25.

My patients and students have various reactions to my announcement — angry, afraid, concerned, and approving. "Do you have a board certified surgeon? You'll look like your husband had beaten you up! Maybe you'll die on the table. Maybe you'll decide to go all the way and close your practice. You don't look like you need it. Oh, why not? Good for you." All of them are grateful that I'm preparing them for the change. It will be seven weeks until we meet again. They are not grateful about that.

JAEDENE
In it together

At the beginning of April, I make the appointment for the only available morning in early summer. I think that no one wants that time because the date is the 13th. But it's Wednesday, and not Friday the 13th. So I decide it's okay for me. I don't want to wait any longer. I want to have it done so that I have the summer to recuperate fully. Life gets much busier in the fall.

When I tell Jill I am having "it" done on the 13th, she tells me her date is the 11th of the same month. We both scream like little girls who are delighted that they will be in the same class.

Jill says, "I didn't think you would ever decide to do it."

"How could you think that?" I ask.

"I thought you were having too much fun with the fore-play."

Yes, it was fun to investigate: to question, look, and compare. But of course I wanted to go for the goal ... to look like a restored, rested ME.

5

What We Worry About

JILL
Facing surgery

ALL I WANT IS TO LOOK BETTER, LESS TIRED, LESS SHRUNKEN AND CRUMPLED. But what if I get punished for being vain and competitive? What if my wish leads to terrible disfigurement? What if I get really ill? So I squeeze in all my annual check-ups. I should be relaxing, and here I am running around to doctors' offices. Why am I compelled to do this? I want to be sure that there are no serious illnesses that should be taking precedence over my face. I'm also thinking that if any of the doctors find something that needs surgery I'll have that done first, and have the facelift because I'm off work anyway. I must be looking for an excuse to have what I want.

For two weeks before surgery I must be off vitamin C and aspirin. Without vitamin C, especially when I'm on an airplane, I might catch a cold and my surgery could be cancelled. What if I get a migraine and can't take anything for it, how will I keep going? What if I get a sunburn or get hit in the face by a tennis ball, will he still operate? What if I mix up the pre-operative instructions regarding pills and antiseptic body wash? What if, what if …

These are the things I focus on, but really I am anxious about the upcoming surgery, period. How will I deal with not seeing for two days and not being allowed to talk for six days afterwards? How helpless will I feel? How will I make sense of my surroundings?

The night before surgery, Jaedene calls to ask if I am scared. No, I'm not. I've finished worrying, and now I'm not afraid. I feel excited, full of anticipation.

Going to the surgicenter

David's taking me to the surgicenter, and I am glad he's with me. During the drive, I run through the What Ifs again: "What am I doing? I may destroy myself. What if I am the first patient to have a facial nerve injury? What if I never again look like me? What if I get my period on the operating table? What if I throw up and burst all my stitches? Will that ruin the facelift? What if I don't like the result? I won't be able to hide it. Will my husband still find me attractive?" No, here's the real thing. I will never look the same again.

Once in the waiting room, I keep looking around me as if I might lose something — a credit card, my glasses. At registration, David stays with me to keep track of my things. What else am I afraid of losing? I'm not afraid of losing my life on the table. I've been close to death and this doesn't feel anything like that. I'm not afraid of anesthesia: it blots out all memory of pain. It's not a fear of death or pain. It's a fear of losing a part of me. Now I have it. It's a fear of being mutilated. That's why I'd be worried about blood being on the sheets.

It's time for him to go. A nurse takes me from the waiting room into the operating area to change into a gown, cap, and support stockings. He gives me a pill to raise my blood pressure because it runs low. The anesthesiologist gives me a tiny shot of local on the vein so I don't feel a thing when she starts my intravenous line. The physician's assistant twists my hair tightly in tiny clumps with rubber bands. How would she manage that if I had long hair like Jaedene?

I go off with Dr. B to get more photos taken and to have him mark up my face with a purple pencil. It looks as if he has drawn in more wrinkles than I already have, like a graffiti artist adding frowns on the face of a smiling woman in an advertisement. That done, I lie down, and the light anesthetic puts me to sleep. I know no more until I wake up coughing.

I have been on the table for nine hours.

*J*AEDENE
Going to the hospital
Getting up at 5 a.m. on the morning of my surgery, I would like to forget the whole thing. My thoughts are partly with what it was like the last time I was in hospital, and they thought I was going to die from the anesthetic. What would be the point of a facelift if I don't live to "show and tell?" There is a moment when I almost back out, but the need to go ahead is strong. Despite my fears, I want to do this.

The ambulatory unit may be fine for Jill, but I am glad that Dr. A does facelifts only in a hospital facility, because I might need emergency medical help if my blood pressure acts up again. I remind Dr. A that this happened before in surgery, and I ask him what he would do. He replies that if it happened during this surgery, don't worry, he would stop the operation. Okay.... But then, WHAT ABOUT MY FACE?!!! How does one look after a facelift has been stopped IN THE MIDDLE!

We enter the lobby of the hospital at 6:15 a.m. There is already a line at the check-in counter. I am starting to shake. I sit down, and Chuck gets in line for me. I close my eyes, trying to pretend I am somewhere else. It doesn't work. I try deep breathing. I really don't want to faint. Somehow, my knees hold me up when my turn comes, and we are led into a small examination room. I am told to change and lie down on the table.

Dr. A arrives, looking natty and cheerful. One of his assistants is with him, already dressed in his scrubs. Dr. A draws all over my face with magic marker, and holds up a mirror so that I can see what he has done. It seems like such a simple and unprofessional way to proceed — just drawing on my face. But I keep telling myself that he knows what he is doing. He asks if there is anything I want him to know. I remind him for the umpteenth time, that I want to look natural, not "pulled." I think of threatening him, somehow, to emphasize the importance of "no pulling," but I decide that threats might not be the wisest choice at this time.

The orthopedic surgeon who will operate on my ganglion arrives. Hearty hellos are exchanged all around. The room is getting crowded. Two nurses arrive. More hearty hellos. Dr. A leaves to change.

THE *f*ACELIFT *d*IARIES

Chuck and I kiss goodbye, and a nurse sticks the biggest needle I have ever seen into the front of my thigh.

Preparing Yourself Emotionally

We know some women who go in for a facelift as if it is nothing. That's not us. We're writing for women who want to know what it's like and who want to face fear and work through it. Read books, talk to friends, shop around, ask the right questions, and trust your instincts. You can come to terms with your experience and learn a lot about yourself, and that helps you through the next challenge.

THE *f*ACELIFT *d*IARIES

6

At Home Like a Baby

JILL, Week 1, Monday at 7:00 p.m.
See no, speak no

SOMEONE IS CALLING MY NAME. A WOMAN WITH A LIGHT VOICE HELPS ME INTO MY WARM-UP SUIT, takes my hand and wheels me down the corridor to the elevator. She walks me over a bumpy path and guides my turbaned head carefully into her car. I feel the car stop and start many times as we finally make our exit and edge along the clogged downtown streets toward Massachusetts Avenue. I ask her to call out the places we are passing — Dupont Circle, the British Embassy, the Cathedral, Crate and Barrel. At last, I am home, facing a long night with a woman I've never seen. I'm told her name is Liz.

David meets us at home. "Okay," he says. "You're home

47

now and I'm right here." He helps us up to the spare bedroom where the woman will ice my eyes and care for my face all night so that we won't disturb his sleep.

I'm not allowed to see for two days and mustn't talk for six. How am I going to manage that? My eyes will not open and my mouth feels sandy like the bottom of a parrot's cage. I'm not in pain, but that's because my face is mostly numb, especially the left side, and on that side the nostril doesn't function. Air can move on the right side of my nose, but actually my mouth is stuck open, so it's not an issue. My bandage is snug, my face is smothered in grease, and I feel hot.

I have to sleep sitting up at 45 degrees. I choose to recover in the velvet reclining chair. That chair felt great for recovering from my previous surgery nine years ago in December. Now it's a typical Washington summer and the velvet makes it too cozy for comfort. I am so hot!

Liz gives me a blissful sip of water and with it one Oxycodone (Percoset) for the pain that might develop as the anesthetic wears off. Saying it's time to ice my eyes, she dips a cotton gauze square in ice water. The edges of the gauze feel like the tines of a fork as they touch my eyelids and deliver their stinging cool liquid. I'm glad when the sting eases off and I'm left with the wonderful coolness.

Liz explains that she will put some special ointment on my face, a pleasant smelling stuff called CX-10. Slowly and gently, she strokes it on with a baby Q-tip. I'm allowed two Percoset every three to four hours, but one of them is enough to send me drifting off. I waken each time she lays the icy gauze on my eyes, lifts off the old ointment with a Q-tip dipped in ice water, and applies more ointment. I'm dismayed to find that it's not morning. It's only 8:30 p.m.

David comes in to check on us. He's holding my hand,

asking me how I feel, and I'm writing my answer blindfolded: "No pain, very tight. And I'm way too hot. I can't bear the heat."

"Okay," he says. "You take our bedroom, and I'll move into the spare room. You'll feel better there."

I go to our bed, propped up on many pillows. I can control the extra air-conditioner there. I keep the room very, very cold.

It seems like hours later, but it's only 9:30 p.m. Now it's only 11:00 p.m. "How will I ever get through this night?" I wonder, as David leaves to go to sleep in the other room. Seeing nothing and feeling lonely, I want my mother.

Lying here isn't painful. I just feel confined in my tight, new face-case, and I'm horribly hot, my face greased up, like a long distance ocean swimmer. But I'm not going anywhere any time soon and I only wish I could get the room as cold as the ocean. I drink, but I have no appetite.

About 1:00 a.m. the skylight fills with light that breaks its way through my gauze eye patches. An engine rumbles and the beep-beep of a truck backing up signals the arrival of the water company nighttime crew. They have chosen tonight of all nights to start work on replacing the neighborhood water pipes. I am so glad that they save the jackhammers for tomorrow. It's irritating, but it's a welcome diversion. This night is so-o long.

Jill, Tuesday
Pill-popping guardians of my healing

Morning comes and David visits. He says my mother survived her laser treatment, but won't know for a few weeks if it helps her vision. I nod to show I've heard, but I can't speak.

Liz tells him I'm doing fine. He says Jaedene called to check on how I am. I write: "Tell her, no pain just tight. Ice stings but soon eases." She's going for surgery tomorrow and I don't want to tell her how time seems to stop. I write, "How do I look?" He tells me I am unrecognizable, like an alien, but he is sure I will be better in a couple of weeks. I want to believe him.

Sally takes over from Liz. They are good friends and they sound alike in the enforced darkness; interchangeable guardians of my healing. Sally has the hard part. One Percoset every three hours has been fine but now it's time to add the antibiotic, the antiviral, and the steroid to the mix. I'm also taking the herb Arnica Montana to help prevent bruising. Sally wants me to have something in my stomach, apple juice, pineapple juice (also recommended for the bruising) broth, yogurt, apple sauce. I have no nausea, and no retching, and yet I throw up (a reflex, Sally calls it). So I'm getting anxious about how I'm going to manage if I can't take the pills. This is the longest day. I talk to myself: "You're doing this in memory of Auntie Dorrie. No one in her right mind could actually choose to do this for herself."

Sally stays calm and offers what she calls "cracker therapy". She puts a tiny fragment of a saltine on my tongue, and it softens there. I find this physically helpful and emotionally intriguing. It's amazing how my whole system seems to concentrate on the edges of the cracker, it disappearing on my tongue, and then the arrival of the next piece and the sensation of the shape of it. But I still can't keep a pill down.

At the change of shift, Sally and Liz work out a new strategy. They use the Phenergan suppository prescribed for nausea even though I have no nausea. They figure out that the only heavy-duty codeine to come in suppository form is

Dilaudid. One of each of those medicines settles me for the night and by morning my stomach is ready to catch up on its pill-taking. They have ordered Hydrocodone (Vicodan) which I will tolerate much better than Percoset. Sally sends out for baby food as the vehicle of choice to get the medicine into me, and I'm thrilled and relieved to discover Gerber's mixed fruit yogurt. It conveys each pill safely down the hatch one at a time every 15 minutes. I feel like a baby who can have only one new food to try each week.

My step-daughter Kate asks to come and visit. She says it's weird that my face is totally unrecognizable under the bandages, and yet my hands are moving just like they always did. She says that I am like a mummy with someone behind me in the bed "doing the hands."

For Sleeping Upright, and Feeling Cool and Comfortable

A firm wedge pillow
Four soft pillows (one for under the knees)
A good air-conditioner
A nightgown that buttons down the front
or slips on and off the shoulders
and has sleeves or a robe (the room's freezing)
4x4 pure cotton gauze squares
A small basin
Baby-safe Q-tips, like Cottoneve baby protector swabs
Vaseline or Aquafor ointment
Arnica Montana pellets 30C
Extra-strength Tylenol gelcaps
Mylanta or Zantac for stomach irritation
Metamucil if medicine shuts down the colon
Kleenex tissues
Sensitive Eyes eye-drops

JAEDENE, WEDNESDAY AT 7 PM
Time to go home

Someone is calling my name. She is telling me it's time to get dressed to go home. I have no intention of moving. I can't see. I'm dizzy. My head feels pushed in from all sides, and I cannot imagine getting dressed, with or without help. She is dressing me anyway and moving me into the wheelchair.

I hear my husband's voice from somewhere far off, and then I am in the car. He doesn't have much sense of direction. I wonder, vaguely, if we will get lost.

We are almost home. I am nauseous. Chuck talks me out of the car and walks backwards as I hold both of his arms and move with short, shuffling baby steps into the house. I feel utterly helpless. I am hurrying, not seeing. He is asking me to slow down. I warn him that I am going to throw up. We make it up the stairs. I am moving by willpower alone.

Now I'm in my room. I sit down on the corner of the bed, throw up into the bowl he is holding, and wet my pants at the same time. He asks if I know I've done it. I know! I HATE it! Thank God Tammy the nurse arrives at that moment.

I hear her talking to Chuck. Gently, she gets me out of my clothes. I don't have a nightgown that buttons down the front. So she puts me into his nightshirt. As my left arm goes through the sleeve, I realize there is a cast on my wrist! That's where I had the ganglion removed at the same time that I was having my face lifted, but I hadn't thought there would be a cast. I hadn't thought, period.

Dr. A had told us that I wouldn't like having the lasered areas on my face wiped clean. "She won't be happy with you," he told Chuck, "and it will have to be done every hour for at least three days."

I wake up each time Tammy cleans those areas under my eyes and above my top lip. But I like the cool gauze pads that are applied first. It is disturbing to me that I can't see her. She puts some moisture drops in my eyes, and they sting TERRIBLY. She tries some salve, and that feels better. I wonder if I will ever see again. I doubt it.

Tammy warned me, a few days before the surgery, that many people feel claustrophobic the first night because of the bandages wrapped tightly around the head and chin. I certainly feel the pressure, particularly under my chin, and I wonder how I will get through the night, until they will be removed at the doctor's office the next morning. I worry, to myself, about how I can even sit up to get dressed. But then the pain medication takes over, and I sleep — until Tammy is doing the wiping again.

There is no real pain from my face or neck, just an unrelenting feeling of pressure and pulling. The pain is in my upper back, from lying in an elevated position. Tammy rearranges the pillows, but nothing works to make me comfortable. I decide that I will have to find a way to be "zen-like" and accept it.

What You Need Most of All

- *A VERY good private nurse for 24 hours, preferably 48 hours*
- *At least one person who loves you enough to tell you every day that you're looking better and it'll all work out well*

7

Getting Off the Bandages

JILL, WEEK 1 CONTINUED, WEDNESDAY
The big one goes

*N*OW IT'S DAY 3 AND DAVID'S DRIVING ME TO SEE DR. B. I'm excited because I'll get my big turban off, all the while thinking of Jaedene getting hers on. It feels good to be a couple of days ahead. It feels horrible to be driven downtown. I curse every speed bump. When I get to Dr. B's office, his physician's assistant Annie takes me into the treatment room. (She's the one who twisted my hair in rubber bands before surgery). She takes the turban off, takes out a few stitches, pulls out the drains on either side of my head (strange, like water gurgling in my ears), cleans my eyes and takes some crusts off my skin. She tells me the good news is — I'm healing beautifully. She gets my eyes open a crack and

I see that my face is purple where the laser has burned me, and green where the ointment is. The bad news is — there's another turban beneath the first one and it still feels tight on my neck! Still, I look less like Nefertiti in the tomb and more like Mata Hari caught in the headlights.

My blonde hair is hidden under the white turban, my nose has become broad, my thin lips are swollen and crusted, and my face is stained brown with iodine. I look like a burn victim. When Kate comes over again, she says my face bears no resemblance to anyone she has ever seen before, but David tells her I look less like an alien today. I'm only glad that he sees me as someone from this planet.

Back home, I'm wiped out. Sally and Liz are GONE. David is striding around my room, monitoring my pill taking, and doing the icing, wiping and smearing routine. It's just not the same. Even the teaspoon feels bigger and harder than before.

I miss my nurses! I miss the soft, slow way they patter around the room. I miss their kind of gauze. The stuff we were able to buy at the drugstore is made of rayon and it feels horrible. They had all the time in the world for me. David has to hurry to get to the office. I try to take care of myself. I check up on his thoroughness with the ointment and the pills, and I'm far too tired to cope with it at all. Not only that, it's ridiculous, because half my face is still numb and I can't tell whether he covered it properly or not. I feel vulnerable and ungrateful. I realize he is hanging on to his work not just to help me pay for all this, but to hold on to his equanimity. I am glad to learn that Sally will come in for one more night after all.

It's Wednesday, and Jaedene is going through her first night, my third. I ask David to take some baby yogurt over to her house. Her husband, Chuck calls to say she loves it. Some mothers say it's bad because it's full of fat and sugar but for mature women with swollen lips and stitches below their gums it's just great. I open my mouth as far as it will go, which is not much bigger than the beak of a baby bird eager for a morsel, try to scoop it off the spoon without hitting the hard edges of the teaspoon, and foolishly push the food away with the tip of my tongue. I feel just like a baby!

The card from Judy that arrives in the morning suggests something else I could feel like: "As you're recovering …" it begins on the cover, "Relax. Put your feet up. Have people bring you things. You know … Pretend you're a man."

jAEDENE, THURSDAY
Bandage off, drain in

It's Day 2 for me, and early in the morning, Chuck goes to row on the river. Tammy gets me dressed. I don't care how I look. Chuck returns to take me to the doctor. Even though I can't see yet, I still have to direct him to the office. We get there and he walks me into the building. I can hear people murmuring, moving out of our way. I have no scarf on my head. I imagine myself looking like a beaten-up conehead, and I have the cast on my arm too! Pathetic. I tell myself that it doesn't matter, there are more important things to worry about, like what could happen to my head and face when the bandages holding "things" together are taken off.

The nurse IMMEDIATELY leads Chuck, who is leading me, into an interior examination room. I am sure she has brought me inside right away because I look too horrible for the other patients to bear. But I am grateful too. Now I can lie down.

Dr. A walks in. He sounds happy. Good for him.

As he removes the bandages, he tells me that Marjorie, our older daughter, called him after the operation to ask how it went. I am touched. I knew Chuck had talked to our daughters and my mother when it was over. There were no plans for any of them to come and visit, but Stephanie, our younger daughter had offered to come and help if we needed her, and had sent bath salts and body cream. I think that, if they had been with me, I would have felt that I had to appear stronger to them, FOR them. I could SOUND okay on the telephone much sooner.

Dr. A is explaining that the drainage tube, coming out of someplace in the back of my head, is still draining and can't come out. A drainage tube? "What does this mean?" I ask. I feel very worried that something dreadful is happening. He assures me that it will stop when it is ready — no problem. But I also hear his surprise at how much fluid has accumulated.

"What have I done?" I ask myself.

Dr. A removes the last of the dressings. He reminds me that he is leaving town the next day and the doctor who covers for him will remove the tube.

No bandages! But the same pressure is still there under my chin! Dr. A explains that the pressure is from the internal stitches. He and Chuck are admiring the line of my chin and the way my neck looks. I am wondering how long I can stand the feeling that I am wearing a bathing cap strap that is TOO TIGHT under my chin.

My long hair is plastered to my head. As we are leaving, the nurse asks if I have a scarf. I don't, so she puts some paper towels on my head. Now I really look gross. But, more importantly, I will have to get dressed AGAIN tomorrow!

For your mouth that can't work properly

- *Gerber's mixed fruit yogurt*
- *A small, smooth teaspoon*
- *Small cans of pineapple juice*
- *Saltines, plain or multi-grain*
- *Dunking cookies: Wheatolo, graham crackers, shortbread, biscotti*
- *Soup that has been through the blender*
- *Scrambled eggs*
- *Corn pudding*
- *Jello*

*J*ILL, THURSDAY
A blur of pills

I'm feeling depressed because Jaedene, who is two days behind me, got her bandage off already — not that her hair looks any good, she assures me, and she still has her drain in. David goes to visit and tells me her lips are swollen, and her face is covered with cream, but her eyes are visible and she is not so red and crusty as I am. I feel jealous and slightly frightened. Why is it taking me so long? I can see a bit with one eye, but the other will not open. David goes to work and the day stretches unforgivingly ahead.

Surprise! My eldest daughter, Zoe shows up on her way to work and stands in the doorway looking away from me. Squinting at her with my one open eye, I see that she looks beautiful and it is a great pleasure to me, but it hurts that she can't stand to get closer. David reminds me that she can't help it. She hates hospitals, injuries, and blood. But here she is saying a guarded "Hi" from the doorway. That's a big step for her.

David's mother decides to visit and calls to discuss her time of arrival in a few days. I beg her to wait another week until I don't look like such a freak, but she isn't fazed. She wants to see David on Father's Day and keep me company. "But I can't talk!" I grunt throatily. "That doesn't matter," she assures me, as if to say that she will do all the talking. I am in a panic.

Day 4 is a blur of pills, face-cleanings, snoozing, and worrying about Grandma's visit. I try listening to books on tape but I keep drifting off and losing the place. I have no idea which characters the reader is talking about or how they fit into the story. The only tape I can follow is Brighton Beach Memoirs because it is short with different voices interacting dramatically, and I know it already. The single reading voice is too hypnotic, or maybe it's the painkillers. Those pills are wild! I keep thinking I see a large person looming over there and another right next to me. I try to push them each away, and realize that no one is there.

Tonight, the whole bedroom turns into a forest. Out of the bushes come a series of dissolving faces. Fish fly out of the top of a man's head. I am flying through the dark undergrowth and taking a canopy tour across the tops of the trees where myriad birds flutter and chirp. This must be what it is like for a really imaginative child at bedtime.

At 4:00 a.m. I am lying awake and I hear my son come home. I call out to him and he comes in. He sits in the darkness, holds my hand and asks me how I'm doing. He tells me proudly about getting a new job and entertains me with stories about his trip to the club where his friend's band is playing. He goes off to bed. Thankful for his visit, I drift back to sleep.

JAEDENE, FRIDAY
No fun house

Chuck has been up and down all night taking care of me. I know he's exhausted. We should have had a nurse for one more day. But the doctor and the nurses had all said that we only needed Tammy until she could show Chuck what to do, and then he could easily take over. She did show him. He's doing a great job but he has a lot to learn. As Jill's husband David says, "It's heavy-duty nursing."

Chuck gets us to the office of the doctor who is covering for Dr. A. I wait in the car while he checks out the length of the wait, and how crowded the waiting room is. By the time he comes back, I don't care. It feels too hot to stay in the car. The waiting room is full, but, this time, I have a scarf. I still hear the murmuring, and someone gets up and gives me a seat.

The doctor says that I am still draining. I feel scared. I think about crying, but it seems like such a useless thing to do. Chuck tells him that my eye has been bleeding. I didn't know that! The doctor puts some drops in my eye, removes a suture, and lo and behold, I can see — sort of. He prescribes more drops, and says to come back on Sunday. Today is Friday. He tells Chuck to measure the fluid that drains, saying that if he takes the tube out now with me still draining I will need another operation. He tells me to go home and lie low.

I have no other plans.

Chuck takes me home and helps me change. I catch a glimpse of myself in the bathroom mirror. BIG mistake. I look AWFUL. It's like seeing a face distorted in a fun-house mirror. But this is no fun house, it's my house, and I won't look again for awhile.

I open a care package with tapes and magazines that my friend Ruth sent. I can't read, but I can look at the pictures in the magazines. I enjoy listening to the tapes of Marlene Deitrich singing in German because I can't follow the words, and so there's no point in trying. David arrives with some more mixed fruit yogurt baby food and a note from Jill, which I find comforting. David tells me I'm looking okay, better than Jill. I'm sorry about Jill, but I'm happy to hear what he says about me. I decide to believe him.

I am exhausted from my trip to the doctor. I am exhausted from the night-time hallucinations of leering people and trees. They seem real, right there in my room, not like dreams at all, and I wake up talking to them. This is in addition to being awakened by Chuck wiping off the lasered areas on my face, or waking myself up to check the time because he's fallen into a deep sleep and maybe it's been too long since he wiped those areas. I realize that dealing with me is like having a new-born in the house.

Jill, Friday
Drug-induced giants

Jaedene tells me in a confidential tone, "I'm having audio-hallucinations." Of course she is. It's hard to imagine anyone actually enjoying these pain pills enough to get addicted. I can't wait to get onto Tylenol, but for now the stronger pain pill helps me to overlook the irritating tightness around my neck and face because it makes me too busy fending off the imaginary giants in my half-awake state to think about pain. I try watching television but it's too big a strain on my only working eye, and way overstimulating. I settle for half an hour of a Britwit re-run that I practically know by heart and can enjoy without having to watch.

JAEDENE, SATURDAY
He must really love me

Chuck planned to row in a regatta in Philadelphia today. I thought I'd feel okay by now. I'm far from feeling okay. I am weak, swollen, and afraid to take care of myself. Chuck and I agree that I can't be left alone. We don't want to burden Stephanie who offers to come home. We consider the nurse. But I don't really want to be left with her either. The weather is awful — wind, rain, thunder. I am thrilled! I insist that it must be like this in Philadelphia too. Chuck says he can't leave me like this. I agree, feeling guilty but relieved.

He is cleaning the lasered areas every two hours now. I tell him that he must love me very much to look at me, clean me off, and still be able to sit and eat with me. He is surprised that I would think that way. I am very grateful to him, at the same time that I'm feeling very sorry for me.

A FEW HOURS LATEr, I have no patience with him, as he tries to rearrange my pillows, and I can't get comfortable, and the drops he's dropping into my eyes keep rolling out, and ... and ... and.

I have been talking to Jill every day. It's very helpful to have her there. She is two days ahead of me in recovery, and she understands how I'm feeling because she has been there too. We discuss baby food, not being able to focus, pressure, unending sensations of heat (are these hot flashes?), mania, denial, acceptance, children, husbands and friends. I regret having told so many people about my surgery. She has told almost no one, except her patients. I should have kept my mouth shut. Yet it's nice to have friends calling. However, I'm very aware of who has called and who has not.

I feel pressured about "showing myself." Jill is taking seven weeks off from work. I am taking less than three. What was I thinking? I will never be ready. But I don't think I'd have a practice to go back to if I'd take seven weeks off. I do feel good about having told my patients the truth about what I am doing. They are grateful for that. I know they must be worried. They know that I will return calls after the first week. I hope I feel like responding by then.

My mother calls to say Hello and asks how I'm doing. I tell her I'm fine. I'm still dealing with her saying I was a jerk for choosing to have this surgery. I don't tell her that it is a big relief not to get dressed today. I still can't stay focused on a movie or even a book on tape. I listen to some CDs. I read parts of the paper, some television, and that's it.

Jill, Saturday
Grandma's coming

It's Saturday and David has left me to drive to Baltimore to meet Grandma's plane. Zoe is in charge of me. She can now approach the bed but she still can't look at me. I feel alone and unprotected from the onslaught of a visitor. I burst into tears — which isn't like me at all — and it isn't easy because my muscles don't move and no tears come out. Zoe does look, sees my muscles quiver, and feels bad for me. She comes forward, actually holds my hand, and rubs my back in a sweet way that lets me regain my composure.

"You must be missing Xanthe," she said. "She's the care-giver child, isn't she?"

I said, "You're doing everything I need and I know it's really hard for you so I appreciate it all the more."

Now David's back and Grandma's here. She looks great. She gives me a beautiful powder compact (definitely for future use) and I grunt an appreciative thank you without moving my lips. She tells me the stories of her bridge friends and her outings, and her visit is turning out to be pleasant, but she can't take the 65 degree temperature. So pretty soon I have my ice-chest all to myself again. She and David go off to a movie with Kate. Zoe stays home to make me some great scrambled eggs. A perfect dinner.

Now I immerse myself in a play-on-tape production of the Brothers Karamazov. Talk about a soap opera! All about male rivalry and murder, blessedly nothing to do with my current concerns. It's not short and easy like Brighton Beach Memoirs, and I get totally lost. When Chuck hears that, he promises to send me his favorite short radio plays of Samuel Beckett. Sounds great. What on earth am I thinking?

David, Grandma, and Kate get home. I feel desperate about having to wait until after their dinner for David to have time to do my face. He tells me that he met Chuck in the drugstore buying no-tangle no-tears baby shampoo and Q-tips for Jaedene. He said he was proud he could show Chuck the baby-safe Q-tips. I hear them on the phone sometimes, like two mothers comparing their babies' progress.

Jaedene, Sunday
Drain's out!

It's Sunday, and I want the drainage tube OUT. I feel its presence is some sort of failure on my part. Chuck measures the contents. GROSS! I don't know how he can do it, but the doctor wants to know.

I get dressed and we go at the appointed time to the doctor's office. We wait 40 minutes. He doesn't show up. We leave our cell-phone number and go home to wait. On the way, we drop off some Beckett tapes for Jill. As Chuck heads for the door, I tell him that I would like to see Jill if she is willing to see me.

What a relief! She looks terrible! I wonder why I can look at her and not at myself.

I realize that I'm feeling euphoric about being able to see and be seen. David's mother is there with Jill and David, all of them looking at me. Their son is not around, but their eldest daughter comes to the door of the room. I greet her, and she says Hi, but I notice that she is averting her eyes.

The doctor calls back to explain that he had an emergency and he can see us now. Chuck guides me to the car, and I sink into the seat, exhausted.

I am afraid of having the drainage tube removed even though Jill told me it wasn't bad. This facelift business is turning out to be one scary thing after another. There is so much that neither Jill nor I were prepared for. We agree that we would rather "know." I say that we should be taping our conversations because they have been helpful to us, and might help others, but we don't do it — because we don't feel like doing ANYTHING.

The doctor is there this time. He pulls the tube out quickly. It isn't bad, and now it's DONE. He tells me I can take a shower and wash my hair. He assures me that the shower will make me feel better. How can I wash my hair? I can't feel my scalp, and I'm afraid of the water beating down on my head. What will it do to my face? Chuck is concerned that I will slip and fall because I'm not steady on my feet.

We are back home, and Chuck is telling me to get up off the bed and take a shower. I reach for his hand to lift myself up, and he pulls it away, saying that it hurts from rowing. I am hurt. I am afraid of taking that shower. I feel vulnerable, and I'm crying as I step into the shower. I refuse the chair he tries to put in the shower stall. I focus on hating him instead of being scared.

My hair is clean! Another accomplishment. Another baby step.

Now Chuck is telling me I should stop taking the pain pills. NO WAY. Dr A is taking half the stitches and staples out tomorrow. I'm staying on the pain pills.

Jill can't help me here. Her doctor takes almost everything out at once, and he doesn't do it for another week.

*J*ILL, SUNDAY
Father's Day visitors
This Sunday is Father's Day. As the mother and the wife I feel I should make it special, but I just can't do much. I ask David how he's doing with the lack of sex.

"Honestly," he says, "I just don't have any desire when I'm babying you and not even recognizing you."

I'm glad he's not frustrated but it's hard to hear that.

Jaedene is going to see the doctor again, even though it's Sunday. I don't get to see my doctor until tomorrow. Jealousy again. The doctor isn't in, so they drop by our house to deliver the Beckett tapes Chuck promised.

Jaedene looks amazingly elegant, in a ghostly sort of way. Her face is a ghastly cream color except around her eyes which are purple, her lips are swollen but not crusty like mine, and her eyes are wide open and one of them is bleeding. Charming. Her head is swathed in an elegant scarf that matches her freshly laundered sepia-colored linen shirt. A length of plastic tubing comes out from under the scarf and ends in the breast pocket of her shirt. Her hand is in a cast protecting her wrist. She looks weird but in a different way than I do. Where she looks like a gaunt and ghostly version of herself, I look like a burned and fattened android. Whatever, she looks ahead of me in progress.

Jaedene reminds me that we are healing at different rates because our surgeons are different, our skin is different, and our faces are different. David is no help. He says that I must have had more extensive procedures because I looked like I needed it more than Jaedene in the first place — which Jaedene says is RIDICULOUS. I remind myself that this is not a neck and neck race (so to speak). I go upstairs to rest.

Jaedene and I both had deep tissue lifts, but our surgeons had different techniques. Jaedene did have a little fat dropped into her cheeks, but I had the fat lifted back up on to my cheeks and secured there. That's why I'm taking longer. In my work as a psychoanalyst, I go for securing in-depth change. I only hope that's the right approach for my face.

I come down this evening ten minutes before Father's Day dinner. The table is not set. Our children are not home. David is in the shower. Can't they do anything without me? Do I have to do everything? I guess that's just the way it's been, and I haven't minded. I feel I should be able to make this a nice dinner as usual, but I have no energy.

When they do arrive, the children proceed to argue and call each other names like I haven't heard since they were in junior high school. David emerges from the shower exactly on time, and pulls the meal together. I can't eat anything but the mashed potatoes and the creamed spinach. End of a difficult day.

Daniel comes up to say Good-night before he goes out for the evening. I ask, "Daniel, what is bothering you and Zoe?" He says, "Don't complain to me about us. Look what you did! You had no right to let Jaedene and Chuck just walk in here, just drop by with her looking like that. I was walking through to the living room and I saw this ghost come in the front door. She looked like the walking dead. It's outrageous. And as for you and her parading around like that — it was disgusting. It gave me the shivers. I mean, it's completely unacceptable."

It isn't just that the children are angry I am not taking care of them as usual. Now I realize how scared they are by the sight of me and how traumatic it is for them. I say, "I'm sorry, I should have warned you Jaedene was coming, but I didn't know myself. I'm surprised by how you feel. You were so good sitting and talking with me the other night. You seemed to be dealing with me well. Are you disgusted about me too?"

"No. That first night when I talked to you at 4 o'clock in the morning, I couldn't see you. I didn't know you looked this bad. The next time I saw you, I could handle it. But Jaedene and you together was too much." He switched to gallows humor: "You were like the walking green mask of the living dead and the unholy abomination of Satan's minions. It looked like the Day of the Dead in here!"

The first week

The first week is mainly about being tired, needing help, and keeping cool. Having your own room air-conditioner is a boon. It's a good idea to arrange plenty of physical help and emotional support. If your helpers can make you comfortable and you can accept your dependency, you can enjoy the pampering. But it's good to fight against it a bit to push yourself to the next stage. You don't look anything like yourself. Helping children deal with that is the hardest thing of all. It's a challenge to you. You look like someone from another climate and an unknown planet, but you think you'll be back to normal in a week. It's going to take longer than that.

8

Showering and Seeing Our Faces

JAEDENE, WEEK 2, MONDAY
The perfect Manhattan

•

*i*T'S MY DAY 6, AND DR. A IS BACK. CHUCK IS OFF WORK
SO THAT HE CAN TAKE ME TO SEE HIM. I'm partly looking
forward to it because I think it will relieve the pressure under
my chin.

The nurses are happy that I'm feeling better. They say I'm
looking good now. They tell me they felt badly for me when
I was last there.

Dr. A begins removing the stitches. It stings. It's disconcerting to hear him working on the staples. He checks my
eyes, and tells me to discontinue the drops. I complain about
looking lopsided. He's not concerned, and assures me it will
be fine. The laser only needs to be wiped three times a day

now! Chuck suggests that I stop the pain pills. Dr. A offers a milder prescription — Tylenol. What good will that do, I wonder? I ask about drinking Manhattans instead. He's happy with that alternative. Not as happy as I am.

I report the news to Jill. She's not had to wipe the laser area more than three times a day since the first two days. She tells me not to worry about being lop-sided. Dr. B has explained to her that the two sides of the face heal at different rates. That makes sense.

I am exhausted from being tense about the stitch and staple removal. That tight-bathing-cap-strap feeling is still there!

Chuck makes me a Manhattan. It is the requisite number of hours since my last and final pain pill. My drink tastes sharp and strong to me, and I sip it slowly. In fact, everything tastes too strong to me. My taste-buds seem to have been affected by the facelift. Even toothpaste has a strong taste, and seems to make my lips swell. The good news is I get to brush my teeth!

Chuck asks if I remember the first night at home. I assure him that I do. Now he tells me that it was frightening to look at me. I looked like I was the victim of a world war, with a fully bandaged head, a bloody eye, and a drainage tube hanging out. I know how difficult it has been for him. I am glad he has had his rowing, but between nursing, rowing, and working, he is exhausted.

By the end of the evening, I am cranky and uncomfortable. There is a "pulling" feeling under my skin, my back is bothering me, and I want a real pain pill. I take two Tylenol instead. Dr. A has given me permission to sleep on my side. My wrist is out of the cast and in an ace bandage that is less cumbersome but leaves my wrist more vulnerable. It stings and hurts periodically. Dr. A says it will take longer to heal than my face.

I am awake for long periods during the night. I know I'm tired. I want to sleep. Chuck is sleeping. I can't call Jill at 3 a.m. to commiserate. Why did I have my face and wrist done at the same time? Also, I have a couple of stitches next to my belly button where a little fat was removed to use somewhere in my face. Those sting. I can't get comfortable. Talking to my daughters on the phone, I laughingly refer to myself as "Mrs. Silence-of-the-Lambs-thrown-down-the-stairs." They don't laugh. I realize that I scared them. I've lost my perspective on what is scary. I talk about stitches, staples, swelling of my face, and blood in my eye, as though they are everyday, mundane occurrences, and people gasp quietly. Their reactions make me feel separate from them. But I am in the middle of something separate right now. That is why it is so helpful to have Jill going through it at the same time.

I pick up one of the magazines from Ruth, and read that women are speaking more openly about having plastic surgery. One woman admitted in print that she had "been to Texas." I don't feel excited about saying, "I've been to Bethesda."

Without the pain pill there are no tall, leering people in the room. I feel really alone.

*J*ILL, MONDAY
Seeing in stereo

Grandma has left for the airport. Jaedene calls to say she got antibiotic drops for her bloody eye and it's much better. She tells me she was scared to take a shower, but then it didn't feel bad because her scalp felt nothing at all! That sounds pretty weird. I'm expecting to be allowed to shower today. I'm off all medications now and I'm excited to be going to the doctor this afternoon for my one-week check-up. I've been getting through this long weekend by imagining the bliss of having the remaining turban removed.

The car ride downtown is no problem this time. I must be feeling better. I hide behind David in the back of the elevator and emerge into the cool of Annie's treatment room. Yes, she is taking off the last bandage. Yes, it is the final one. So why does my neck still feel so tight, or as Jaedene puts it, like I have a bathing-cap strap under there all the time? My spirits sink. Annie reminds me it's tight because it's meant to be. Meanwhile she suggests 2.5 mg of valium for the next two weeks to ease the feeling of tension. And she takes out the stitch that's been annoying me at the corner of each eye! Both eyes now open an equal amount so that now I can see in stereo. Annie says that I can use Vaseline instead of the CX-10 ointment with the smell I am beginning to hate. I'm thrilled when she lets me take home some of the gauze I love. It's come to this!

I look in the mirror and the face that looks back at me is a lot better than last week, though still android. It's so unlike me that I imagine they took off my head and switched it with the next patient's! No, that's definitely my dirty blonde hair, matted down and poking up in places. The good news is — I can brush my teeth, take a shower, and wash my hair with the usual shampoo. The bad news is — I can't blow-dry it because the staples above my ears will burn.

At home, I try to brush my teeth. The bad news is — the usual toothpaste burns my lips and the brush won't fit because my lips are stiff. The good news is — Zoe gets me a children's toothbrush and toothpaste — a green-with-sparkles, glow-in-the-dark Barbie toothbrush and pink bubble-gum paste. I feel like a kid, ready to jump in the shower. A minute later, I decide against it. I'm too exhausted by the simple effort of brushing my teeth and trying to make my eyes work together.

Meg comes to visit. I've known her since she worked as a nurse in Edinburgh before we both came to the United States. Meg offers to stand by while I shower — which she has done for me before. She nursed me through my serious illness five years ago, and she's the best friend anyone could ever have. Compared to her, Jaedene is a new friend, someone with whom I love sharing my thoughts, but I can't imagine her tending to me in my bathroom. Even with Meg's support, I can't get up the energy to get in the shower. I'm scared I'm going to faint in there. Meg leaves to pick up her daughter, and I drift off again until the phone rings.

Kate calls and asks, "Is your face still numb?"

"Not entirely. I now feel occasional, odd, spontaneous sensations in my cheeks like a spring uncoiling or twanging or water trickling, and a tickling feeling as if there are hairs inside my chin. My lips are stiff but not quite as crusty."

"I heard you couldn't eat corn at dinner and that you were wishing for corn pudding," she continues. "I've got the recipe here for you."

The recipe! Why couldn't she make it for me? (I don't say that). I know I look and sound better but I feel lousy. Not until evening can I make myself get out of bed and into the shower.

This shower feels great! My scalp does feel the shampoo after all. It's nice to see my hair is still there even though there seems to be less of it. Looking at myself in the mirror as I comb above my ears, I notice a small round bruise on my right cheek near my mouth and pretend it is a dimple. I think my face is moving slightly and I see an expression like a week-old baby's windy smile, or did I imagine it? The woman in the mirror has two open eyes, albeit they are merely slanted slits. She looks quite friendly though weird. She is nothing at all like me. Even my hair looks wispy because I can't use the blow-dryer. My scalp feels like the net backing of a wig, but who would buy a wig with such a sparse amount of hair?

I fall into bed exhausted.

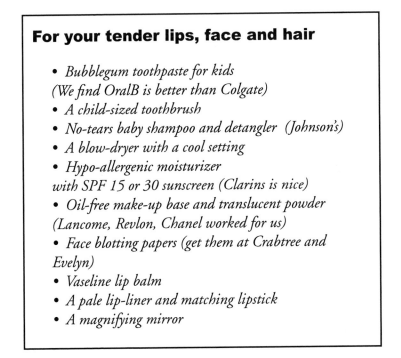

For your tender lips, face and hair

- *Bubblegum toothpaste for kids*
(We find OralB is better than Colgate)
- *A child-sized toothbrush*
- *No-tears baby shampoo and detangler (Johnson's)*
- *A blow-dryer with a cool setting*
- *Hypo-allergenic moisturizer*
with SPF 15 or 30 sunscreen (Clarins is nice)
- *Oil-free make-up base and translucent powder*
(Lancome, Revlon, Chanel worked for us)
- *Face blotting papers (get them at Crabtree and Evelyn)*
- *Vaseline lip balm*
- *A pale lip-liner and matching lipstick*
- *A magnifying mirror*

JAEDENE, TUESDAY
A lump-of-clay day

I don't hear Chuck shut the door as he leaves to go rowing at 5:30 a.m. I wake up when he comes back. I can feel my face, wrist, and stomach. I take the Tylenol capsules. I don't believe they do anything for anyone, but I need to do something. I'm still taking an antibiotic and an anti-viral pill. I don't have to take Arnica any longer. My legs feel rubbery as I walk to the bathroom. I force myself to look into the mirror for more than a quick glance. I still look pretty disturbing.

Believe me, it's difficult to wash your face when you can't feel where it's being touched. My face feels like someone else's, and I don't recognize its terrain because of the uneven swelling in unexpected places.

Chuck brings me the baby yogurt and coffee before he leaves. I get on the phone to Jill.

Jill is talking about the people she sees around her house every day. I say that I like being alone. But I'm starting to feel socially phobic for the first time in my life. The only person I see is Chuck. I don't want anyone to see me. I don't feel like holding up my end of an in-person conversation yet. I'm worrying about being able to meet with my patients in a week and a half.

I take a nap. Somehow it's easier to sleep during the day. It feels safer. I don't wonder if I can sleep long enough, as I do when I'm hoping to sleep through the night.

Chuck comes home, exhausted. He falls asleep. I don't. I feel like I'm wearing earmuffs and swim goggles. I watch television for awhile, but it doesn't hold my attention, and at 11 p.m. I get on the computer for the first time since the operation, and check my email.

Jill, Tuesday
Dishing about our doctors

I wake up feeling more energetic and hopeful. Jaedene asks me to watch a television program called The View, because it features women like us talking with Barbara Walters about what's happening to them. They laugh and joke at each other's expense and if you can't see them too well it doesn't matter. It's highly entertaining but the ads are too much for my eyes to take. I really didn't realize how many bursts of light come out of ads to keep our attention. I keep wondering which of the women had facelifts and if I'll turn out like one of them.

I call Jaedene back. She tells me she heard that the surgeon she consulted in New York is the one who did Barbara Walters' face. I ask, "Why didn't you choose him after all that, and, I've never asked you this, but why didn't you go to Dr. B? After all, you got us his name, you saw him before I did, and you said you liked him."

"I liked the guy in New York too," she replies, "but I decided I didn't want to recover away from home. I chose Dr. A because I had seen several people he worked on and thought they all looked natural. I thought he would listen to me better than Dr. B. You know surgeons can be arrogant, pretty detached. I knew Dr. A's wife from our book club and she helps out in his office. I'm glad I had that."

So that's it. I had judged Dr. B, not by whether I liked him or whether he listened to me, but by whether I could listen to him. I wanted to know if the things he said to me made medical sense and seemed to be appropriate to my face.

"What do you think of Dr. B?" she continues. "I liked

him, but he's eccentric."

I find myself defending my doctor. I say, "Eccentric? No. He's creative. Arrogant? No. I think he's deep in thought. Cold and detached? I don't think so. He cares how I'm doing. Sally was his operating room nurse for twenty years and she loved working for him."

"What do you know?" Jaedene says. "Post-surgical days 9 and 7 — and we're discussing our doctors."

I suppose it is inevitable: a little competition.

I go to clean my face and I can't find the soft cotton swabs that Annie gave me. I have to use the horrible rayon ones from the drugstore. It feels like the end of the world. I go downstairs for dinner but I still can't chew the steak or crack the corn kernels. My day ends with mashed potatoes and peas. That's what I feel like.

JAEDENE, WEDNESDAY
What the butler saw

It is Wednesday. I think about what I was doing last Wednesday and am grateful I have come this far. I'm expecting the cleaning woman today. She doesn't know about my face, and I'm figuring out how I will tell her before she sees me. I hear the door open, and when she walks into the front hall, I call to her from upstairs. I explain what I've had done, and then walk halfway down the stairs and sit down. She looks at me and laughs with relief. She says that if I hadn't told her, she would have thought that maybe my husband had beaten me up. She asks if there is anything she can do for me. I only wish there were.

It is ironic that today I am beginning to feel impatient with the swelling and recovery, because there is nothing that

I want to be doing. But I'm STARTING to think of things I SHOULD be doing, like going through the piles of papers on my desk. I tell myself that I have plenty of time to take care of that. I consider working on a photograph album.

My great-aunt calls. She's 89 now. She had a facelift 35 years ago, and then some work done after that. It is heartening to speak to her. She is supportive and excited for me. I tell her that Chuck and I will be down to visit and show her the results in about six weeks.

Even though I want to hear from my friends, it is tiring to keep speaking on the phone. Also, I'M getting bored with hearing myself describe how I am.

9

At Home for Callers

JILL, WEEK 2 CONTINUED, WEDNESDAY
The lost swabs and the Fellini lunch

•

*I*T'S BEEN 10 DAYS SINCE MY SURGERY, AND I STILL FEEL
LIKE A MASHED POTATO. I check my messages. There's one
from Jaedene: "I'm glad to hear that losing your swabs was
the worst thing that happened to you today, although I certainly do understand. And that is why I think that our conversations are much more interesting than those on television
because they would help others who have to go through this
after us. A happy thought has just occurred to me for today.
You and I never have to listen to — or even read about —
those skin-formula, line-firming ads again because they have
nothing to do with us. We have taken care of all that for
ever!"

I find my swabs! They had fallen among Samuel Beckett's radio plays (exquisitely poetic but way too weird for me in my present state of mind). I get up, shower, and dress. I wipe my face with the swabs, and grease my face and clean my eyes with baby Q-tips. Lo and behold my eyes now function together and I can keep my glasses on. This is a much better day. I'm back in business.

Jaedene goes to Dr. A again today to get more stitches out. Again she and Chuck drop in on their way there. The back of her long hair is out of control and her face is a mixture of green and purple bruises. But her eyes are clear, and only one side of her mouth is swollen. How can she feel like wearing a smart blue linen shirt, when I am in the same warm-up suit I've been wearing for days now? I tell myself I'll emerge out of this cocoon on Monday when I get all MY stitches out.

Jaedene, Thursday
The chin-strap feeling

Chuck is off work to take me to Dr. A's office. I don't want to drive myself, because I feel rubbery on my feet.

We are taken into the exam room right away, not because I look hideous as I did last time. Dr. A gets right to work on removing stitches. He's talking as he does it, which works well for me, giving me something to take my mind off of it. It stings, but it's not bad. FOR SURE, I have decided, the 'chin-strap' feeling will be gone NOW. Dr. A's wife, my friend, comes in to say "Hi." I watch her looking at me, and I see that she doesn't seem freaked out in the least. So my face must seem okay, but my knees feel weak.

We stop at Jill and David's on our way home. I'm happy they invite us to stay for lunch. It's my second social outing.

My eyes are bigger than my mouth. I can manage one scallop, two forkfuls of salad (I couldn't manage salad before today) and two forkfuls of cantaloupe. Jill has one scallop cut in tiny pieces and some pineapple juice. David and Chuck, looking outdoorsy and unbelievably normal, are merrily eating away. The contrast is hilarious. Jill starts barking, her form of laughter at this point. I look around and laugh too, mine sounding like snorting, because we can't open our mouths wide enough. It's like a scene in a very strange Woody Allen or Fellini movie. We are all sitting and eating as though our situation is absolutely natural. It's Thursday afternoon, none of us are working, and it feels like these are moments outside of time. David and Chuck are looking at us as though we are insane. We are, a little.

When I get home, I go directly to bed, exhausted. It's been 9 days, and the 'chin-strap' feeling is STILL THERE. Will it be there for THE REST OF MY LIFE?

*J*ILL, THURSDAY
Encased in a mask

I'm at my computer again. I'm finishing up an article on the death instinct and keeping a facelift diary — one about death and the other about looking younger. A total coincidence?

Jaedene calls to say, "Thanks for lunch."

I say, "I've been thinking about what Dr. A told you regarding the chin-strap feeling going away when the last stitches come out. I only hope it proves true for me. I've told David that if I still have that feeling in four weeks, I won't be able to travel. The thought of being cooped up in a plane seat with my face trapped in a tight mask is more than I can stand. I'll want to jump out of my skin and out of the plane as well. I wish you were coming. I'll have to deal with how I'm doing all by myself."

She says, "We are lucky to have had each other going through this. It's been so helpful to know what you told me about the face healing unevenly. Or just to worry together about whether it's okay to feel so swollen or frozen or like we are living in a mask. How many women get that?"

I say, "Probably not many, though they could if they talked to friends about it. Or if there was a book that really told it the way it is, up close and personal. A lot of people are pretty secretive but they would rather be talking like we are. Now that I've been open, I'm getting emails from women who want to think about having their faces done. It's been great talking about it, instant peer therapy.

"My biggest fear is that I won't look like myself. When I confessed that to Zoe, she said, 'Well, I hope you won't look like yourself. Isn't that what you are paying him for?'"

"Only a daughter!" says Jaedene. Then getting back to the matter at hand, she continues, "On Monday, I'll really get the last of my stitches out. Then I get to meet Dr. A's make-up artist who has her own stuff to cover my bruises."

"On Monday, I get the rest of my stitches out too, so we'll be even," I say.

I can't believe I said that.

For dinner I'm going to have an excellent small steak, very rare, and some fresh corn pudding. Jaedene says, "What about a DRINK?"

JAEDENE, FRIDAY
Feeling depressed

I watch The View on television. I talk to Jill, and it's noon already. Jill is much more energetic than I am. She is up at 7:00 a.m.; she's going to the office; she's writing and editing on her computer; and she's DRESSED ALL DAY. Never mind that she looks like shit. I am lying in bed like a lump of clay, staring at the television or gazing out the window, talking on the phone, thinking about doing my desk or my photo album but not until tomorrow, feeling that I will never be energetic again.

I speak to Jill. She is exhausted! She's beginning to think she is overdoing it and maybe there is something to relaxing. I am SO relieved to hear that. I am the "voice of relaxation."

I'm home alone! I decide to tackle the photo album. I talk myself into it by giving myself permission not to clean off my desk first. I can do the album in bed!

My friend, Marie calls to ask if she can come over for a short visit. I saw her soon after her facelift, but she was OUT AT A RESTAURANT. She was in much better shape than I am at this point. Even so, Marie will be a good choice as the first outsider to see me because I won't feel self-conscious with her, and maybe she'll inspire me to leave the house.

Before I know it, between phone calls and the album, two hours have gone by. My left leg has gone to sleep from being in the same position, and I haven't had lunch. I haven't sat up this long since the operation. I consider skipping lunch, since it's downstairs and I'm tired again, but it doesn't seem like a wise thing to do. It's already 1:30 in the afternoon.

I heat up some soup, and I am looking forward to the baby yogurt. I can't open the jar! My wrist isn't strong enough, and I'm afraid of hurting it. I feel really frustrated. This is a big thing in my day at this point. I give up on the yogurt, and return to bed.

The phone rings again. A friend calls to say that she has "outed" me about my facelift to another friend whom I hadn't told. At first I feel annoyed at her, but then at myself.

Why didn't I tell the second friend? How reasonable is it to expect someone to keep this secret? The fact is that most people will probably guess when they see me anyway. But it's another loss of control. I can't make my face heal any faster, I can't stop people from talking to one another, I can't open the yogurt, I can't have my energy back. I feel depressed.

Jill, Friday
Beyond tired

Jaedene calls. Both of us are still in bed at 10:00 a.m. This seems to be taking far too long.

I confess, "I overdid it again at the office yesterday. Then I was awake much of the night, feeling uncomfortable, unable to get cool. Finally I remembered to take the valium and that helped. I've got to pace myself better today."

"What the hell were you doing in your office yesterday anyway?"

"I'm writing, I'm sending off a paper to a journal, and most of all I'm enjoying how cold it is there. And I want to get back in there but I feel stuck."

"That's the difference between us," she says. "I will be glad just to wash my hair, use the blow-dryer on cool (thanks for the tip) and maybe, maybe, and only if I feel like it, spend forty-five minutes on my desk. But up to now I'm still in my nightgown. Take it easy, and I'll talk to you later." She sounds assured, sensible, taking care of herself, not washed out like me.

Kate calls again, and I'm still in bed, sorting through some bills. "I've lost the recipe for the corn pudding," she says. "Can you read it back to me?"

I had scribbled it on something. Where is it? The plumber's bill floats up to the top of the bedcovers and on the back of it, miraculously there is the recipe. I read it back to her.

Kate asks me, "Did you hear from Dad about Chloe's latest lost tooth?" (Chloe's her 6 year-old daughter, and, No, David hadn't mentioned it.) "It fell down the drain and she was in tears. I thought of taking the drain apart and so I called Dad to come over with a wrench. He said, 'Taking a drain apart is a big deal. I know what to do. Put her on the phone.' Chloe sobs, 'Poppa David, my tooth's gone down the drain and now I don't have it for the tooth fairy.' He goes, 'Sweetheart, I'm sorry your tooth's gone, but here's what you do when that happens. You draw a picture of it and put it under your pillow. The tooth fairy will be happy with that because she gets lots of teeth and hardly any pictures.' Chloe goes, sniff, sniff, 'Okay,' sniff, ''Bye.' Chloe hangs up, and then Dad says to me, 'Sweetheart, this is a lesson in loss. It'll be okay. And I go sniff, sniff, 'Okay,' sniff, ''Bye.'"

I've lost my old face, and like Chloe I don't know what I'll have to show for myself. And I can't make a picture of my face. It could spook the tooth fairy.

Getting back to the recipe, Kate says, "I've decided the thing to do about the corn pudding is to make it for you. I'll bring it over this afternoon. See you later."

YES! Now I feel I can go to my computer.

Later Jaedene calls back. "There are people lining up waiting to see, believe me, they are thinking about it, checking it out on me first. I look like a horse's head and I'm wondering what on earth I have done to myself. It's so good to tell someone that. Marie called and she'll be here in twenty minutes — and I can't deal with it. I'm not ready. I'm exhausted. I just want to stay in bed."

I feel taken aback at this change in Jaedene's confidence. She seemed to be zooming toward recovery and now she sounds as tired as I was this morning and as upset as I was a few days ago.

"Jaedene, this is Day 10 for you. Remember Day 10 was my day for getting over the slump, and even then I slipped back the next evening. You get to wash your hair and you feel you should be fine, but you're not really. After surgery, you feel damned tired, you feel better, and then you slip back. It takes time. Take it easy and enjoy Marie's visit. Tomorrow is a new day. I'll talk to you this evening."

Jaedene, same day
Marie from the WWHHPS

I haul myself from bed to get dressed. There is no chance that I will look attractive, so I go for "comfortable." At the appointed hour, Marie rings the bell. She hugs me, and tells me I'm looking well, considering. I can tell that she means it, but I feel self-conscious. She has brought me some gifts, and it's fun to get them. I give her all the details about me, and she relates them to her own facelift experience. I realize that when she was going through it, but I had not, I was not privy to the same information that she is sharing now. I am now part of a secret sorority of sorts: WWHHPS ... Women Who Have Had Plastic Surgery.

It's time for Marie to go. I return to bed. I feel defensive about being tired. Marie isn't tired, and Jill isn't tired! Competition again.

*j*ILL, SAME DAY
Feeling uneasy and guilty

There is an uneasy thought pressing at the back of my mind and I squash it by going to my computer. The drive is crammed with illustrations I can't clear. A buzzer sounds and I get the on-screen message, "This program has performed an illegal operation!" Quite apt! I shut down.

The uneasy thought comes into view. I am having surgery for purely cosmetic reasons while my husband's eye needs attention, my mother is losing her vision, Chuck should have had his cataracts done, and Catherine is having chemotherapy again. Jaedene and I had serious surgery that meant we lost organs. Do I feel guilty about this operation, which is not exactly necessary, and is that why I feel so shut down? Absolutely.

*j*ILL, SAME DAY
Marie's visit continued

Suddenly there is a knock at the office door. It's Marie now coming to see ME! I ask her how she managed to go out the second week. She says Jaedene was wrong. It was the third week, when she could cover the bruises with make-up. When she had her facelift, Dr. B wasn't using laser, but even so the swelling took a long time to go down, and for a couple of winters her cheeks felt sensitive to cold. I'd found talking to her helpful before surgery because she had had the same doctor. Now I realize that she hadn't told me everything.

"No, I didn't," she agrees. "Women can't tell everything. You have to pick and choose what parts to tell. Don't worry. You'll be so pleased a few weeks from now."

Why do women have to pick and choose? They don't talk about the details of their facelifts, just as they don't talk about sex, and mothers don't explain everything about childbirth. They don't tell what really happens, how it feels, and how long it can take. They believe that no one will do it if they know the truth. We question that. We think it's better to be prepared and to be brought into the community of women.

Jaedene calls again. "I feel okay with you and David, but other than that I now know I am definitely not ready to see people. And it had nothing to do with Marie. It's me. It's the way I am today."

"You're having a down day, like I had earlier this week. I've been amazed at how well you're doing, even though you've been alone all day, whereas David and the kids are in and out to see me."

"I don't mind being alone," she said.

"I know that's true, and it's not that I'm with people all day. But moments of human contact help. We've had that on the telephone, and Wednesday we had a great visit. All the same, we've been a bit manicky, don't you think? And now we've both crashed."

I was glad to hear her laugh. "We've been manicky, you're right, and today has been a sunless day and I don't like that. It's not a bad day. It's a more realistic day. Never mind, here is Chuck with my Manhattan and some of Kate's corn pudding. Things are looking up."

JAEDENE, SATURDAY
Planning movie night

I'm feeling better today. Jill and I agree to rent a movie and have a pot luck dinner at her house. We discuss redecorating her living room. This gives me a reason to look through all the design magazines that Ruth sent. I find a picture of a living room I think Jill will like, and I feel that I have accomplished something. I'm looking forward to socializing, and decide I will put on makeup for the first time.

JILL, SATURDAY
Forgetting about movie night

Mum calls early to see how I'm doing. She's been confined to the house with a flare-up of a knee problem and her friend Betty has had searing chest pain. They've been talking together like Jaedene and me. Betty was alarmed when she felt the chest pain. Her first thought was "It's my heart!" and her second thought was "And I just had the back of the house painted!"

If I get to be Mum's age, I hope I'll still have Jaedene. I hope we'll still have our sense of humor to get us through. Mum still hasn't told any of her friends, not even Betty, about my surgery. What is that? Is she ashamed of me? Or is she the guardian of my own secretiveness?

I'm still in bed when Jaedene calls. She reports from an article called "Scalpel News": "It says here that a study of 79 plastic surgery patients showed that those who had the group support of other patients as they recovered did better than those who recovered alone in private suites." See, there's scientific proof that we are lucky to have each other. And it's proof that I'm right when I say that we should share our diaries with other women, so that they can have someone too."

She moves on to advising me how to re-decorate my living room. She's definitely back on form. We agree to get together this evening with David and Chuck. I'll reheat a curry that I have in the refrigerator and she'll bring rice. I suggest the movie "What Women Want," a title that fits our theme and a fun story pertinent to our situation. She suggests dinner at 6 and home by 9.

By noon I'm reading emails and writing a report. My glasses keep slipping down my greasy nose and obliterating the print. My brain doesn't want to work. I think I'll take a walk and relax until it is time for the movie. But I start on the report as usual.

Before I know it, it's quarter to six. Jaedene and Chuck will be here in fifteen minutes. I don't bother to change because I can't use make-up anyway. I go to get the heavy pot of curry from the back of the refrigerator. I remember I'm not supposed to bend or lift. Suddenly it all seems TOO MUCH.

Jaedene and Chuck arrive looking great. She's moved on from grease to moisturizer, her hair is under control, and she's wearing lovely linen pants, a silk sweater, and high-heeled black patent mules. I'm still in the same old warm-up suit, with the greasy, purple, android face, and the glasses slipping down my nose. Partly I don't care because I don't feel like myself anyway, and partly I feel embarrassed to have made so little effort. She actually looks like herself, but her color is greenish and her eyes are tired. She's worrying about a ripple that she sees on the side of her face and scars that are too far below her eyelids instead of along the lash-line, even though she's been told that it's done that way to spare the lashes. The hell with her. I look like an android.

I can't see well enough to pick at the details. It's because she looks so nearly herself that she sees them. My points of difference are so enormous I'm not looking as closely. What unites us is the worry about what we have done to ourselves. How will we turn out?

JAEDENE, SUNDAY
From slump to clean slate

It's Sunday. Chuck has been rowing everyday. It's his way of dealing with the emotional and physical stress involved with the facelift. He tells me again how upsetting it was to see me the first night. It's taking time for him to get over it. Clearly, it frightened him.

I remember I haven't finished my desk. I'll think about it tomorrow. There is a feeling of competition with Jill who never seems to stop working. No! I WILL clean off my desk, go through my files, and take on the photo album. Two weeks before the surgery, I spent two days cleaning out closets. Now, everywhere I walk in the house, if there are a few papers, I look through them and throw things out. I'm accomplishing something. There is something going on here: cleaning up, cleaning off, a clean slate, a clean face ... a facelift!

Jill and I talk on the phone, and agree that we were both exhausted by the movie evening — sitting up for three hours and keeping up the conversation. So, as much as we both wanted to socialize, we found that it took a lot of energy. We still can't open our mouths fully to eat, or smile, much less talk.

I have tried to forget about my wrist. I don't even like to see the incision, since I can see the thread that runs through the stitches, and I don't like thinking of ALL the stitches running around and through my scalp, face and neck. But my wrist reminds me it's there with some sharp pains every now and then. And speaking of stitches, tomorrow, Monday, I go in to see Dr. A, so that he can take out the rest of the stitches and the STAPLES. I'm feeling nervous.

I actually return to the photo album and FINISH IT.

As a reward, I decide that I will tackle a small piece of steak for dinner.

Jill, Sunday
Sunshine and reflection

Jaedene's been planning to go back to work late next week. How will she sit in a chair keeping up her end of the psychotherapy conversation with her patients hour after hour? She's re-thinking her schedule and canceling a seminar. Oddly enough, she's explained to two of the people in the seminar why she'll be absent but she hasn't told the others. For her, telling is a matter of who she feels close to.

I don't care who knows (they're going to know soon enough anyway), but I notice I'm inclined to avoid the word facelift. It sounds so superficial. I catch myself saying, 'I'm having face surgery' as if that will avoid my being taken for a superficial person. Using this euphemism for facelift is my version of outwitting the forces of prejudice in myself. But I spend money on clothes and hair, and even more to preserve my teeth, so why not on the face that I wear every day? There's a lot to deal with here, and I'm glad I gave myself lots of time to get my strength back.

I want to spend the cool part of this beautiful morning with my face in the shade of the magnolia tree and my body in the light sun, but I can't work it out. Even in the shade

I am worrying: What if I get a sunburn, or what if a mosquito bites my face? I know I am being paranoid, but Jaedene understands. I spend the rest of the day indoors, in neutral gear, willing the time to become 1:00 p.m. on Monday.

The Second Week

The second week is about coping with necessary bursts of activity, tiredness, and anxiety about how long it's taking to get back your energy. You must go into the shower, get yourself dressed, and go to see your surgeon. You feel anxious about letting the nurse or doctor touch your face and take out the next stitches, because you can't believe it's going to be so easy. Then you lie in bed all day. You still don't really want to see people and so you look for things to do, which keeps you entertained but exhausts you. You feel one-dimensional. It seems to take for ever to reach the day you get your last stitches out.

10

Out Come Stitches, and Out We Go

i HAVE AN APPOINTMENT WITH LESLIE, DR. A'S SKIN SPE-
CIALIST IN THE OFFICE. We will discuss makeup to cover
the bruising that is left, and any other makeup ideas she may
have to disguise the fact that my top lip is swollen and so is
my face. I've put on my regular dark lipstick. Leslie suggests
I use a light color. Immediately the proportions of my face
seem to improve and my mouth looks less witch-y. She puts
some cover-up on the bruising, and we both agree that the
stuff I have at home will work just fine. She adds blush, and
I look better, still in a distorted kind of way.

Chuck joins me, and we wait for Dr. A. Chuck is reading
a magazine. I am simply sitting and thinking about what is
to come.

Dr. A is happy with the way I look, and goes on about the business of removing stitches and staples. At one point, he is taking longer on one spot. He exclaims, "Here are your screws". MY SCREWS!! "Yes, you had these two titanium screws in your head. They are quite expensive." He shows them to me, and I tell him that since they were in my head, I want them. I'm going to put them in the silver box with my daughters' baby teeth and my IUD. Chuck isn't saying a word. Dr. A is admiring my chin line and pointing it out to Chuck. I am still thinking about having had screws in my head. Jill has them too, but hers will remain PERMANENTLY.

Dr. A announces that he needs to remove some fluid from my forehead. He says, "It will feel like a mosquito bite." I don't believe him. I am right not to. It feels like a big bee sting, and I'm glad when it's over. He asks if I want to see the fluid. I DON'T. He shows it to Chuck. Chuck is still pretty quiet. Dr. A says we should have an appointment again in two and a half weeks. I am sitting up, feeling woozy. I'm very happy that Chuck is there. Later, he tells me that the needle looked pretty big, and he didn't watch the removal of the screws, and he has a lot of confidence in Dr. A. I make the next appointment, and we walk, slowly, to the car.

When we get home, I fall into bed, and take a long nap. The 'bathing-cap-tight-chin-strap' feeling remains.

*j*ILL, MONDAY
Not on your head

I've been awake since 5:30 a.m., filled with anticipation. This is the day I get the stitches out. I get up, shower, and go to the office for a couple of hours before my appointment.

I dress in a safari suit with a wide-brimmed hat and a long scarf, ready to make an expedition. Because this is the day the new water pipes are actually being laid, my car is parked way up the street. I walk to it briskly, feeling energetic. I arrive at the doctor's office early. Glancing at a magazine in the waiting room, I realize that my old prescription sunglasses are no longer effective as reading glasses, but I pretend to read anyway. I'm trying to avoid talking to the woman who, while waiting for her friend, is asking all the patients what we had done and trying to get a look behind our scarves.

Soon Annie takes me into her treatment room and removes all my stitches and staples. She says they will pull, but they don't bother me at all. As she snips away, I tease her about leaving me some hair please, and she says seriously, "The follicles are fragile. So don't fight with any tangles, but if you lose hair, don't worry. It'll grow back in four months, eye-lashes in three." She tells me to stop using the Vaseline on my face and move on to moisturizer. I ask her if I can exercise. "Yes," she says, "Walking on the treadmill slowly and lifting light arm weights." Hearing that, I ask what she thinks about having sex. "I think it's a great idea," she says. "Just don't you be the one to stand on your head." As if ...

She and Dr. B are glad I'm healing nicely, but they are concerned about the lower corner of my eyelid, which is being pushed out by some gel-like tissue inside it. He gives me steroid drops to use and asks me to take a break from the computer for half an hour four times a day to bind my eyes with a head bandage stretched over gauze eye pads. Enforced rest for me?

Back home, I wash my face and put on some moisturizer and then try the cover-up make-up, first the green stuff, then the colored base. The result is awful. I look as though I'm sweating through a layer of greasepaint. I swear my pores must still be oozing Vaseline. I feel depressed at dinner and my crab cake is just too spicy. Eating it feels too hard to manage. So does everything else.

Jaedene is sympathetic. She has already had the steroid eye-drops and her eyes are better. She thinks I should let my skin clear before using the make-up.

"What did he say about the ripple?" I ask.

"He said my skin was puckering along the line of some internal stitches and as soon as they absorb it will be gone. Nothing to worry about. I decided I have to forget about all this and get on with doing my desk. Tomorrow I'm getting on the treadmill for ten minutes. But right now I'm exhausted. I still don't feel ready to be the object of scrutiny and I'm canceling my appointments until next week."

"I'll miss these chats when we're back at work," I say.

JAEDENE, TUESDAY
Sorting the BIG pile

I am happy that yesterday is over. But I can no longer put off the job of finishing cleaning my desk. I check in with Jill. She has been writing, editing, emailing, faxing. I think she said something about feeling tired again. I hope so!

I bring a BIG pile of papers from my desk and drop them on the bed. Now I HAVE to get on with it. I start going through them. They make me aware that I will see a patient in only three more days. Jill thinks I need more time. I assure her that if I feel I do, I will call the patient and reschedule. I DON'T know, at this point, how I'm going to be able to do it. But it has been two weeks, and I'm looking less swollen each day.

I decide to try 15 minutes of slow walking on the treadmill. Dr. A has told me its okay. I do it. I feel fine. I spend most of the day working on my files, sorting through the BIG pile of papers.

I have agreed to go out and have lunch with two friends tomorrow. I tell Jill I still feel weird because I have the bathing cap strap feeling under my chin. I'm worried about people staring at me, because my upper lip is swollen, I can feel extra fluid in my forehead, and my face perspires. I think I still look freakish, and my friends might be put off by the way I look. She knows it's very important to me that I go. It will get me ready for going to the office and seeing my first patient the day after tomorrow.

Hints on physical activity

- *At 2 weeks, walk slowly on the treadmill for 5 minutes*
- *Work up to 30 minutes on the treadmill*
- *Start with hand weights*
- *Have sex if you feel like it*
- *At 8 weeks, do push ups and anything else*
- *If your face swells, stop*
- *Wait two weeks and try exercise again*

JILL, TUESDAY
Still a weirdo

Up early, eyes already wrapped with the steroid drops in place, showered and hair freshly blown dry, I attack the make-up problem with greater restraint. I use the palest lipstick I own and even so I resemble a clown. I mustn't use eye-makeup except on my eyebrows. The only problem is finding them. They've always been blonde and I've lost some eyebrow hair. Without contact lenses I can't see them and since my skin is numb I can't feel where to draw the lines either. Whatever, my pencil-work looks better than nothing. My eyes are still android and I still look like a freak, but I have energy and I feel optimistic.

Jaedene has more energy too. She drove herself to see me and she had already been on the treadmill for fifteen minutes. Compared to her, I still look weird.

"Have you bandaged your eyes yet?" Jaedene prompts me.

"Yes, twice yesterday and once this morning," I said. "And I didn't mind it at all. Each time I just fell asleep."

"And what is that telling us?" she says, teasing me about working too hard.

"And how are you doing?" I say, changing the focus.

"My eye-stitches are still there, but my ripple has gone. My mouth was looking more normal this morning too, but then I made an interesting observation. After I brushed my teeth, my lips became more swollen again. I think that my toothpaste is too irritating."

"Me, too," I agree. "That's why I've been using kiddie toothpaste."

"You might have mentioned that to me," she says forlornly.

For your first outing

- *Good, large, dark, outdoor sunglasses
to shade you from the sun*
- *Good, large, light, indoor sunglasses
to shade you from people*
- *SPF 30 sun-block
(check the expiration date)*
- *One broad-brimmed hat*
- *One nice long silk scarf*

"I'm sorry," I reply. "I didn't know you were having a problem with brushing. My usual toothpaste was killing me and that's why Zoe got me the children's toothpaste, and she got me a child's toothbrush because my mouth won't open all the way."

"That's very important information and should be made available for people like us," she says. "Our conversations really should have been recorded. The way we're talking is part of opening up the topic."

I tell her, "Like Mandy and Ellie called me to ask how I was and how I chose my surgeon. They were telling me all the people they've taken to their appointments and various choices of surgeons. Ellie's thinking about something for herself, but she says she'll probably decide by not deciding."

"Oh please," says Jaedene. "I'm sure she already had her face done. And he had his eyes done. Aren't you glad you've got me to help you with your naïveté?"

Now I remember Ellie's parting shot: 'So when does David go under the knife?'

I have to go. There is a raccoon digging up my impatiens.

Jaedene, Wednesday
Out to lunch

I am afraid to exercise AND wash and dry my hair AND go out for lunch. I'm afraid I will be too tired to hold up my end of the conversation. So, I skip the exercise, and focus on getting ready to go out. I wash and dry my hair, and lie down for 15 minutes. I'm tired from feeling anxious. I put on my own lighter moisturizer today, hoping that it will sink in, unlike the stuff from Dr. A, and I won't have the greasy look, even though I know nothing sinks into recently lasered swollen skin. Using my moisturizer makes little difference and mine has no sunscreen in it. So I have to go out with my skin shining, which I hate.

My friends come to pick me up and tell me that they are amazed at how well I look. They expected MUCH worse from my description of myself. They are very happy for me, and call me "Dr. A's poster child." I am feeling shaky, and my legs feel rubbery. It's very hot and sunny out, 100 degrees, and I'm worried about the sun shining on the lasered areas of my face.

We go to a restaurant where we have never been and don't expect to run into anyone we know. I look around to see if people are looking at me. I don't take off my sunglasses. No one is looking at me, except my two friends. We discuss my face for another few minutes, and move on to other topics. I feel as if there is a girdle on my face, earmuffs on my ears, and goggles on my eyes. It takes effort to focus on the conversation. Inside, I'm telling myself to relax, that these are people who care about me and are wishing me well. Susan reminds me, "It isn't ALL about your face." She's right. I calm down.

I can't eat as much of my lunch as I would like because the amount of food looks HUGE compared to what I've been eating, I still can't open my mouth fully, and my hands are shaking.

We finish lunch and have a 10-minute walk to the car in full, hot sun. I'm relieved to get into the car. They drop me off. I want to be inside the house, alone. I get back into my nightgown and lie down.

Jill and I conclude that having lunch out was a wise decision — for ME. Of course SHE hasn't gone out yet, and SHE isn't returning to work for another month.

JAEDENE, THURSDAY
One day to go
I have my first inkling that it's not that I don't look too great, but that I don't look TOO bad. I am turning the corner, and there's still time to change my mind about tomorrow. It's a Friday and I'll only see two patients, then rest all weekend.

JAEDENE, FRIDAY
The BIG Day
It's Day 17 and that's the day I plan to go back to work. I am supposed to go to a seminar on infant observation, but I'm anxious about the observation of ME. Because I look swollen, I would have to explain to all the members in the seminar what I have been up to. I'm not ready yet. One thing at a time. I should be at a committee meeting later this after-

noon. I'm skipping that too. I'll go to the next one. I want to look better than this when they see me for the first time.

I put on some cover-up makeup. It doesn't really cover up the bruising, even though there's not a lot of it to cover. I wear something red to take some attention from my face. FAT CHANCE. The good thing is that the patient I'm seeing works in a hospital setting, and has seen A LOT.

When the time comes for the first appointment, I walk to the waiting room, call the patient's name, and walk back to my office. The patient comes into my office, looks at me and says she feels relieved. I look better than she expected because I don't have bandages or obvious scars. But she notes that this is the first time I have not faced her as I greet her in the waiting room. I want her to see me for the first time in my private office setting. She says she thought about me all day on the 13th. I ask how she felt during my absence. She begins to speak about her past few weeks, and tells a bad dream about someone running away from her. She asks if I have read the book Veronika Decides to Kill Herself. My heart sinks. Oh great, my absence has been too hard for her. She explains that it is the story of a young woman who realizes that life is only what she makes it. Thinking she is going to die, Veronika begins to let herself and others know more about how she feels and what she thinks. She decides she desperately wants to live, and she does! The fictional Veronika gives me a good feeling about how the patient has done without me after all.

Another patient complains that her previous therapist intruded on her therapy by having more than one facelift, and more than one breast augmentation, during the course of the treatment. Silently I say to myself that I'm glad I didn't have anything done to my breasts. At the same time, the patient tells me she's relieved that my breasts don't look larger. She's also pleased my face looks good and my eyes look young. She asks for the name of my plastic surgeon. Then she picks up the thread of her own narrative. I'm glad it isn't all about MY face.

Still, I have to make an effort to focus on what she is saying. I feel that somehow my brain has been affected by the surgery that I know was confined to my face. Am I mentally and physically strong enough to be doing this work now? I think so. It's just harder than usual, being too aware of how my face feels. Yet, it is also a relief to be back, to be doing what I normally do. The operation is OVER, and I have made it back!

JILL, WEDNESDAY, THURSDAY, FRIDAY
Maybe for you, but not for me

It may be over for Jaedene under three weeks but it isn't over for me. Check in with me in another two months.

Jaedene and I have been so preoccupied with our faces it's easy to forget that other people aren't. We've been dealing with our fears and discomforts by thinking of each other almost as one. We both want to get beyond our faces and find more in our lives than that. Only she is ready to do it. She's taking her face out into the world, starting with her girlfriends to season herself for the first meetings with patients. She asks again if I'll join her next week. I hate to disappoint her, but I just don't feel ready to go out for lunch.

I still don't look like me. I've been dealing with not seeing myself in my face by perusing Jaedene's face for signs of herself emerging, and I've not been disappointed. I envy her that she looks so natural, so like herself by now. But my face is a different matter. I feel as if I have five faces and they're always changing.

There's the young face that I've grown out of and don't want back; the old face that I was headed toward and wanted to avoid; the recent face that I have now got rid of even though it wasn't awful; the 40 year-old face that I'd like to see again; and the face that will eventually be mine that I can't quite imagine yet — a face continuous with mine and yet better than mine was recently, and that's the face that eludes me. Will I ever look like me again?

SATURDAY
Jaedene gets busy and I chill

Chuck is away rowing all day Saturday. Jaedene is writing about her recovery. I feel as if I've handed the task to her, she's picked it up, and now it's my turn to relax.

David has the house full of faculty and students for a seminar this weekend and the rest of this week. It's quite taxing and I spend my time hiding in my office or asleep in my bed, but I do surface to have lunch with the faculty because they are my colleagues too. I've been looking forward to seeing Yolanda (of the wonderful facelift), but I don't have the energy to take her out to dinner. She totally understands. She reminds me that at six months, her face was still triangular, her eyes were pulled from the sides, and her cheeks were swollen. She knew that people felt puzzled by her looks, and not until a year had gone by did she look entirely like herself again.

The Third Week

By the third week, you have more energy. Driving brings independence. Seeing yourself in the mirror is still shocking but having the use of cosmetics lets you hide the temporary signs of damage and distortion. You can put "a good face on it" as you attempt to rejoin the world. This week is hard because you still don't look like you and you think by now you should, even if you have been told otherwise. You have to deal with continuing tightness, numbness, itching, swelling, and redness. Not everyone heals at the same rate, and some of you have a harder time than others, depending on what you had done and how your tissues heal. You may feel anxious about seeing friends, but you can do it.

11
Complications

JILL, WEEK 4, MONDAY
The car dies

I
T'S DAY 22 FOR ME, AND I TAKE MYSELF TO SEE DR. B, DRIVING DAVID'S CAR because the children at home prefer my car, the Explorer. Dr. B says that my eyes are slightly better. So now I can stop binding them with gauze and bandage, but I have to press on the lagging outer corner of the left eye 100 times a day. I can do this.

On the way home, the alternator dies in the middle lane at a traffic light. I can deal with the car. I can slide it in neutral back into the right lane and park legally. The nearest garage is only a block away, and there I can call for someone to pick me up. But I have to walk in the bright sun and talk to a person who will look at my hot face and take my name. I feel for a moment the kind of panic I felt when I was stuck for two hours in traffic on the Beltway late in the ninth month of pregnancy. I should have taken my own car.

I can deal with this. Lucky I brought a scarf and hat.

That would kill me

This evening we deal with Jaedene's crisis (on her Day 20). "Guess what?" she says. "The next big step in this process is — what must be a yeast infection. I've never had this kind of burning and itching before, and it's driving me insane. This thing is going to kill me."

I say, "I'm sorry. You got it from the steroids and antibiotics you had to take for the facelift."

This is not pleasant to discuss, but this is one complication of having a facelift that no one else will talk about. Jaedene says that the only good thing about it is she has totally forgotten about her face.

JAEDENE, MONDAY
Diflucan does the trick

There is something really embarrassing about admitting to having a yeast infection. I confide in my daughter, and she is totally matter-of-fact. She says not to waste my time with any over-the-counter stuff. "Go straight to one dose of Diflucan," she orders. My plastic surgeon (who isn't surprised) immediately hands me a prescription. It's over! I should have checked with my daughter first.

*j*ILL, WEDNESDAY
Independence Day, not

It's July Fourth and I am not going to see the fireworks. Too bad, I've got the costume covered with my blue eyes and red and white face. But Jaedene's going. She's got her make-up on and she's OUT AND ABOUT. I'm huddled at home thinking about make-up. I realize that if you cover redness with green make-up, you then need a much darker, browner foundation than a white-skinned person could ever imagine wearing. I decide to forget about my face, and paint my nails red, white, and blue.

THURSDAY
Do I have to?

Jaedene wants me to come for a glass of wine with her girlfriends. Oh, do I have to? I think it's important that I do this for HER, but she thinks it's important that I do it for ME. I think she doesn't realize I've had company in the house all week. They leave this afternoon and I'm looking forward to relaxing with the full run of the house to myself. Jaedene asks how I look. I tell her that I don't look too bad today. I can see a glimmer of myself. Even if it's only an expression at the inner corner of my right eye, it's something to hang on to. I finish another article. Working is something to hang on to as well, because at least that feels like me.

FRIDAY
Wining with Jaedene and the ladies

I do join the ladies for wine. I drive myself with my hat brim pulled down over my eyes. Judy, Barbara, Catherine and Susan are there and I feel comfortable with them. They say I look wonderful, which simply can't be what they are thinking particularly if they compare me to Jaedene who has on eye make-up and looks like herself, only better than before. I still look nothing like me, and surely they are wondering, as I am, if I ever will.

Home again, my face starts burning and twanging, and I am in for a rough night.

Jill, Saturday
Another opening, another show

My face looks redder today and I don't dare go outside again. I stay in bed until noon reading the paper. It's amazing how long it takes to actually read the paper. I wonder how people find the time to do that every day. By lunch-time I venture out and sit under the umbrella in the garden and a double layer of sunblock SPF 30. It's pleasant today. I'm glad I'm here.

I call Jaedene to thank her for the wine gathering. Reluctant as I was to accept, it was helpful to get me out there. I'm preparing myself for the sociability that will be expected of me on our trip, ready or not.

Sunday
Totally wrinkle-free

I enjoy a run to the store and I survive shopping for our upcoming trip. I am looking for clothes that claim to be wrinkle-free — like my face.

I get on the treadmill at 3 miles per hour and stay on it for 25 minutes and then lift arm weights for 10 minutes. It feels so good to move around again after weeks of being sedentary. The exercise gives me an appetite and I eat a whole lot of tabouleh. The sudden increase in food gives me a stomach-ache with alarmingly severe cramps that send me to bed with a heating pad at 4 o'clock. Another medical complication.

Jill, Week 5, Monday
Let-down

I call Dr. B to find out the time when he will check my eyelid. Not one appointment left! I must wait until tomorrow. Now I know the full meaning of disappointment.

Tuesday
The eye has it

The corner of my left eye is gradually firming up and I must keep doing the exercise of pushing on it 100 times a day. I can push open the lids now and so I get my lenses in. That feels like a triumph. Now I can wear the lightly shaded sunglasses that let people see my eyes but not closely. I feel much less like an alien, but I still look nothing like me. My skin is not too purple and I can hide the red with my usual concealer. No more of that weird green stuff.

I notice that I've got my physical energy back. Today I cleaned up, did errands, and started packing.

Wednesday
Upset with Jaedene

My manicurist says I look younger, but she wouldn't have recognized me if she hadn't seen my name on the book. My hairdresser is on vacation, but that doesn't matter because I can't cut my hair since I need it to cover my scabs. I can't color it because the color could irritate them. So I'll go off on a trip with a new face and straggly, graying hair. To tell the truth, I'm hiding from my hairdresser because I know he didn't approve of the facelift idea. He thought I'd lose too much hair and that I'd become addicted like some of his clients. I don't think there's much chance of that, but I have to admit my hair does seem thinner. I don't want to hear him say, 'I told you so.'

I drop by Jaedene's to say goodbye. She tells me she talked to Dr. A about my recovery and he said, " ...." I don't listen to what she says he said. I can't believe she did that.

I tell her I am upset. I haven't talked to Dr. B about her, about how much faster she was healing. I'd been told it would be eight weeks before I was recognizable but it was hard to be patient and keep faith. That's why I looked to her for support, but I wasn't looking for a second opinion. Now I am sure she has told him how worried I am about how unlike me my face is, compared to how natural she looks. (I envy her that).

Looking so unrecognizable seems to me to be a private worry I shouldn't be conveying to other doctors. I need reassurance, but I want it from my friends, my husband, and Dr. B — not from some other doctor. Jaedene tells me that our doctors will be seeing each other in a few weeks when they both go on a mission. It is okay for us to talk about them, but it doesn't feel comfortable to think that they might talk about us.

Jaedene says she'll really miss me. I know I will miss her. I wish this bad feeling at the point of separation would go away. As if to comfort me, she tells me that Dr. A said in a few months I would look wonderful, but this does not make me feel wonderful or even hopeful. It only confirms my suspicions that she has revealed to him my distress, and that somehow it might get back to Dr. B as a complaint (one I don't want to make) rather than as an anxiety.

My upset underlines the loss I feel at the parting of our ways as we both go off. So that's what I am really upset about. Losing her. So she mentioned my recovery worries — so what?

THURSDAY
Losing Jaedene

Jaedene is sorry she upset me. She makes a point of telling me that she hasn't told her doctor my name. But I am still mulling it over. Why am I stewing about this? After all, Jaedene and I are writing our deepest feelings to share with the world. So what is this? Here lies a not-so-small island of secrecy and shame on my part. What's it all about? I think I've got it. I must be pretending that if only I looked like myself, then no one would know I'd had anything done.

Twists of the Double-Edged Sword

You look WONDERFUL!
I can see you're still swollen
     You look so much YOUNGER!
         But it was so wise to leave those lines in
You look NATURAL!
         But I can't see you've had anything done
You look GREAT
Now dye your hair a darker color
You look TERRIFIC!
But therapists don't usually have facelifts, do they?

The Fourth and Fifth Weeks

This is a time of moving forward and slipping back. You feel you should be able to do everything but you can't. Your face is still taking a lot of emotional energy. Complications may arise in other parts of your body you don't want to have to attend to. You begin to feel anxious and impatient. You want to work and see your friends, but you may not be totally comfortable with your appearance or with their reactions. Waiting for the final result really does take time. Some of you will find it preoccupying and depressing. Humor helps. As your face continues to change, you have to re-learn how to do your make-up every week.

12

Out and About

*n*OW THAT SHE LOOKS GOOD, JAEDENE IS TALKING ABOUT WHAT IT'S LIKE TO HAVE HER NEW FACE. But I'm still looking a bit weird. She's streaking ahead, and I feel I have lost her. I won't be speaking to her for a couple of weeks because I'll be out of town at a meeting, which will be a vacation too.

I don't mind flying, but this time I'm afraid that my face will feel hot and tightly strapped onto my head, the way my body usually feels in an airplane seat. Fortunately, the plane is cool, the movie is gripping, and I forget how tight my face is.

Checking into the hotel, I'm embarrassed about my greasy face.

*J*AEDENE, FRIDAY
The voice of plastic surgery

We are visiting friends in New York. They are excited to see "the face." I'm starting to feel that my face is an object. The husband, who compliments me on my face, won't let her fix the neck she's complained about for years. His attitude is complicated by the fact that his sister AND sister-in-law have just had their faces done in two different states. And they ARE now in different states: His sister-in-law has recovered quickly; his sister has complications. By the end of the day, the wife declares that she wouldn't have the courage anyway. I start to counter that. Why am I arguing with her? Because she sounds like my mother. Not only that: For all my complaining, I know I look better. I want that for her. But no, I don't have to be "the voice of plastic surgery."

That evening we see a group of friends. The men are immediately complimentary. The women are happy to see me, but seem to be studying "the face." The husband compliments me on my face. The women ask what it was like to have it done. I tell them, and I try to go on to other topics. Except that the facelift has been my sole preoccupation for weeks, and I realize that socially I'm a little out of practice.

*J*ILL, SATURDAY
The nicest thing

Friends who are also attending the meeting arrive at the hotel and look around for me. I hate that moment of recognition of non-recognition. We go together on a subway train that is so crowded that I'm afraid of my face getting bashed. I feel embarrassed and I hide my head. Carol understands immediately and relates: "When my friend had her face done she wouldn't go out to any restaurant because she was all bruised, but I said I didn't care what she looked like, and so she came over to my house for dinner. She was much more bruised than you are. And she looks GREAT now."

That's probably the nicest thing I'll hear today.

SUNDAY
Worse than ever

The days have been cloudy and chilly, but every night at 2 a.m. our sixth floor hotel room heats up. I wake up with a hot face. I throw open the windows and toss off the bed-clothes. Eventually I get to sleep again, and it's hard to get up in the morning. My eyes are swollen, and so I have trouble getting my lenses in. I rush through my make-up. Oddly, in the tiny elevator, there is a lighted mirror and I see that my concealer has left streaks on my face under the make-up, my eyeliner is smudged, and my eyebrow pencil has left a thin harsh line.

It's so weird to be a person who had a facelift in order to look better and who now looks worse than before. This state is supposed to be temporary, but I'm full of doubt. And I do have "chookie cheeks." except that they aren't squishable. I'm starting to brood on whether Dr. B put implants in my cheeks without telling me. My face is just too full, too tight, and too hot to believe. Will this ever be over?

WEEK 6, TUESDAY
It's raining

I'm actually happy that it is raining and so my face stays cool and doesn't feel as tight. I keep catching a glimpse of my unfamiliar face, mirrored in the city shop windows. Who is she, with those slanted eyes and enormous cheeks reddening where they swell below the eyes? I imagine I'm part of a face-altering witness protection program! When friends want to take a photograph, I look for Lesley and hide behind her big hair so as to cover the left half of my face, the side that is the most swollen. I imagine that with only half of me visible I won't look so uneven.

At night in bed, I don't have to look at my face, and I feel more confident knowing that David can't see it either. But I still can't lie on the side of my face because it feels as if I'm wearing headphones. I can't lay the side of my face on his chest because his chest hair feels unbearably tickly. That's a loss to me. I didn't realize that I use the side of my face to connect with him. David told me that he didn't realize how much he looked at my face and needed it to connect to me. In view of that, it's remarkable that he can hold on to his faith in the process of my recovery.

WEDNESDAY
Whining and dining

I'm losing interest in keeping this diary. Who is it for? Jaedene isn't here. Now her face is well on its way and I'm wondering if mine will ever be the right size and shape. I feel impatient and preoccupied. I hate the way my face is taking me over. It used to be encouraging to share the small changes. Now I'm simply whining.

I want to go to sleep, and wake up a month from now, feeling like me again. David doesn't understand that I want a break from people, from so much make-up, from having to make such an effort to get over my discomfort with how unlike me I am.

That bruise I imagined as a dimple weeks ago has come back, only now it really is a dimple in the middle of my right cheek and a weird ripple has developed near my right eye. I remind myself that the ripple Jaedene reported a few weeks ago has disappeared.

I have to rest my face the way I might put my feet up. It gets tired of smiling, talking, chewing, and being hot. And when I rest, it twangs and twizzles. It has to have time to itself in the cool and in the dark. AND SO DO I.

THURSDAY
Making up in the elevator
I can't see to put on my make-up in the bathroom. So I'm using the lighted mirror in the elevator while riding down to the lobby. Sometimes I ride back up again to the sixth floor if the mascara doesn't go on well the first time. The good news is the elevator is slow and the long ride lets me do a perfect cover-up job. The bad news is I end up looking fake.

JAEDENE, FRIDAY
No one noticed
BIG day in Washington. Two professional meetings and a dinner party. Only one person in each of those groups "knows" about the facelift, and no one says anything about it. Susan was right. It's not all about my face. Do I want it to be? I have to stop myself from announcing the "news." NO ONE SEEMS TO HAVE NOTICED. Yet, I still have an interesting, fun time! Has my life returned to "normal?" Do I want it to?

SATURDAY
His lips are sealed

We are guests at a Washington dinner party. We have great food and lively conversation with our host. When I call to thank him the next day, he tells me that another guest could not believe I was the mother of adult children. I cave and tell him the secret about my face. He assures me his lips are sealed. Too bad mine aren't.

JILL, SUNDAY
Your wife isn't with you?

Now I'm picking up a rental car. The photo on my driver's license is so unlike me I imagine being accused of stealing the car. Help! It's a stick shift. As I press my foot against the clutch, the driver's seat releases and I shoot forward face first into the windshield. I exchange the car for an automatic, but I can't turn in my face.

At a reception, there are many colleagues I haven't seen for a while. Dave recognizes me, but that's because his wife Shelley has warned him. Most of my friends have to be told that it's me under that face. Some of them aren't fazed, like Joyce who says, 'Oh yes. I did that 10 years ago. It'll turn out fine.' Betty, the most outspoken, asks, "What have you done to yourself?" Barbara doesn't even see me. She says, 'Hello David. Your wife isn't with you?' And I'm standing RIGHT NEXT TO HIM.

I HATE this.

JAEDENE, WEEK 7, THURSDAY
You didn't need it

Chuck and I visit my mother and my great-aunt. My mother and my older brother pick us up at the airport. They are eager to see me and my face. My mother keeps saying that I didn't need to improve it. It's flattering to hear this once, but I soon find it annoying. After all, it's now a done deal. Then a woman at the pool says I look too young to be her daughter. If I look too young to be my mother's daughter and too young to be my daughters' mother, where does that leave me? My brother and I joke about it. We agree that I'm now his "much younger" sister. But he also speaks of all the women he knows who have that pulled look. We don't laugh about that.

It's strange to be in Florida and not be sitting in the sun. Even with sunscreen with a sun protection factor of 45, I feel anxious when I'm not under an umbrella. For the first time ever, I'm hoping that there will be some rain, or at least some serious clouds.

FRIDAY
Fish out of water

I don't sleep comfortably, and I'm missing my routine. Usually I enjoy not having a schedule. But, there is no schedule for when my face won't be numb and swollen, and so I want one in other areas of my life. I need to know what I CAN count on.

I'm not too happy with the heat. I'm feeling it more than ever in my life. The facelift has really altered my body thermostat. I swim some laps. I'm not wearing a cap, but I STILL have the bathing-cap-tight-chin-strap feeling.

There have been shark scares in Florida, and so few people are venturing into the ocean. But it looks so-o-o compelling. I want to go in, but I stop to think about it. A shark attack could really mess up my recovery.

SATURDAY
Lonely with the sharks
To hell with shark attack, I'm going into the ocean. There are a few other people in the water, and I swim out toward them. Just in case. The waves carry me, and I feel relaxed and free. If only I didn't have to worry about the sun. Now I'm feeling very alone out here. Of course, "here" isn't just about the ocean. It's about here in my mind — the way I see myself, the way I feel when others are looking at me. And Jill is still away.

JILL, SATURDAY JULY 28
More than I can chew
We meet up with Dave and Shelley at a pool. Their polished bronzed bodies seem more in place here than my white one with the shiny red face. Shelley tells me she had a dream the night before we arrived. In her dream, she was looking for me, but couldn't find me, and so she kept asking every woman if she was Jill, and no one was. Shelley knows she was worried about my seeming strange, and she's glad I don't look as weird as I think I do.

I move off into the shade under an umbrella, a tree, a sunhat, and suncreen. Even so, I have a hot red face by afternoon. In the evening, I put on lots of make-up, so much that I'm a cross between glamorous, fake, and weird. We join Shelley and Dave for a big dinner, a lot of chewing for an easily tired face.

Eight weeks is coming up and I've lost all hope of looking like myself when I go back to work.

JAEDENE, SUNDAY
Looking good and staying that way

I had a mental picture of myself before the surgery. I looked different every day depending on my mood. I knew, even a week after the surgery, when I could bring myself to look closely in the mirror, that there was a big improvement. But, I was not prepared to see it so clearly as when I reviewed the "before" pictures at Dr. A's office.

Is that what I really looked like? The lines look deeper, the puffs puffier, and the bags baggier than I ever imagined. But I am looking from a different perspective now.

What worries me is that there is no way to stop Mother Nature. I remember as a young woman I'd have a perfect hair day and I'd wish it could stay that way forever. I can't freeze my face the way it is today, and I don't want to go back where I've been. So, I guess I WILL have to get involved with the moisturizers, and the treatment creams that I said we would never have to think about again, and the sunblock — now more than ever.

JILL, WEEK 8, TUESDAY
Let's face it

Flying home today, I'm reading old New Yorkers. One of them has a cover picture of a woman in a bathing cap. It's called "End of the Voyage." The image reminds me of Jaedene and the bathing-cap-chin-strap feeling she used to speak about. We wouldn't call that the end of our voyage. At least I'm past that now.

I think about how the sight of me will affect my patients. There's bad news and good news. My face still gets greasy even with light moisturizer and oil-free make-up BUT I can camouflage the shine with powder or face-blotting papers. My left cheek is swollen BUT the swelling is diminishing. The tops of my ears are still numb BUT the lobes are fine and I can wear earrings. My cheeks have red streaks BUT I can hide them. My nose looks broader than it did and if I try to pull the nostrils in, they go out instead BUT I won't do that in the office.

There is some dragging down of the left corner of my eye, BUT it's less and the ripple has smoothed out on the right side of my eye. I can't wear lenses because my left eye feels as if there are hairs inside it and the skin below my eyebrows is swollen BUT I can camouflage that by not wearing eyeliner, using a light-colored concealer stick instead of shadow, and wearing my eyeglasses. Different parts of my forehead are tender from one day to the next, the left side of my forehead and the bridge of my nose have wrinkles, and my face twangs in isolated flashes BUT no one else will know that.

My scalp feels tight and bumpy, not like a wig any more — more like a well-used football helmet — and it itches and gets goosebumps in a heavily airconditioned room BUT cortisone mousse helps, and if I don't scratch it no one will tell anything about my scalp. My hair has lost volume and texture and I can't use color because I'm not completely healed BUT the gray hair is blending in with the blond.

My upper lip is still swollen in the middle and I still can't give a full smile BUT in my job I'm rarely called upon to smile; so that's not a problem. My teeth seem smaller in my new face BUT I'm absolutely sure that the set of my teeth is the one thing in my face that hasn't changed a bit.

The weirdest thing of all is that the teeth I look at now seem to belong to someone else.

Bottom line is, so does the face.

Jaedene, Wednesday
Jill's back

It's my Day 50 and I've just heard from Jill. I'd been assuming that she was having a great time, while I was getting used to working again and continuing to focus on the physical and emotional aspects of "THE LIFT." I had no idea her healing was taking so long and that the trip was hard for her. I felt jealous of her "vacation," but I was relieved that I wasn't traveling far from home. I felt that I could only deal with so much, and there has been too much to date, for me — working, treating medical complications, discussing the impact of my face, coping with exhaustion, traveling, and worrying about how my daughters will feel about the finished product.

Jill, Wednesday and Thursday
How my patients react

I'm back at work, and Jaedene calls to ask how my patients are doing at the sight of me. All of them are concerned about whether I'm in pain. Other than that, their reactions are all across the board. Some think I look good but different. Surprised that I look younger, one of them is missing my wrinkles. One is afraid that I will stop caring about treating him. Some can't see that I've had anything done because there are no scars or bruises and my face doesn't look pulled. Some of them are stunned. They feel as if they are telling their intimate thoughts to a stranger. The only way they feel it's me they're with is to connect to my eyes and my voice.

Being told that I look younger is weird. The swelling makes it seem as if I have got back my baby fat. I got a new face too much like the one I was relieved to lose earlier, and I lost the old face I had. I share my patients' feelings about the loss of my familiar face. I'm not in any pain, but looking unlike me and waiting for my face to settle are the hardest parts of my recovery.

The eight-week anniversary of my surgery is only two days off. Jaedene's already starting to write about what it's like after a facelift. It's not "afterwards" for me yet.

The Sixth, Seventh and Eighth Weeks

You really FEEL like yourself again, but not all of you will LOOK like yourself yet. Comparisons among you breed envy and guilt. The self-questioning continues. The symptoms continue. If you still can't look in the mirror and see the person you think of as you, you are dealing with an assault on your identity. This is a hard time.

JAEDENE, THURSDAY
A little more like herself

It's Jill's Day 53 and at last she looks a little more like herself. More of the swelling has gone down, but she's not looking ENOUGH like herself yet ... and I am wishing she was farther along, for both our sakes. And now, David is starting ... They have more energy than we do.

13

Husbands and Friends
Taking the Plunge

JILL, MONTH 3, FRIDAY
My Day 54 or
David's Day 1, and I can hardly look

I'VE FORGOTTEN ALL ABOUT MY FACE, BECAUSE DAVID IS
NOW THE PATIENT AND I'M THE NURSE.

Yes, men have face surgery too. David is having his eyes
done to correct the extra folds of skin closing in on his eyes.
He had no interest in doing this until I had my face done. He
could imagine the likely improvement in me, he trusted my
surgeon, and therefore he decided not to wait as his father
did until his visual fields were totally restricted. "I only hope
you don't think I'm competing with you," he says. Is he wor-

ried that I'll look better than he does?

David has had only his eyes fixed. He hasn't had a facelift and he hasn't had laser treatment, because in our society loose neck skin, wrinkles, and jowls are more acceptable on a man than on a woman. So his recovery will be easier than mine was. Even so I've booked Sally to help him through the first four hours. I plan to nap while she's at our house, recover from my jetlag, and be prepared to take over from her with ice and gauze to see David through the first night.

I go to get him. David is lying down. His eyes are swollen shut. He is coughing. He looks totally out of it. Why does he have a huge bandage on top of his head AND under his chin when he only had his eyes done? It's to protect the stitches in his scalp and hold in place the drain suction pack that sits on top of his head like a can of tunafish. I know that, but I think the worst. He looks like he's dying. But the nurse gets him up to stagger into his clothes.

When he returns, he feels his way into the wheelchair. He feels squeamish and the nurse gives him a choice of saltines or tiny graham crackers in the shape of teddy bears. He chooses the teddy grahams and I have one too. Those are good. Why didn't they tell me about them? I look at David more closely. He is shaky and slow. His eyes are visible now, and already one of them can open a bit. They are slanted, swollen and purple. One of them is bleeding down his cheek. I feel for him. I'm so glad I saw Jaedene's bleeding eye and I know it is nothing to worry about. I get him into the car, and we have an easy drive home because it's not yet rush hour.

Sally calls to say she has to work late. She cancels! Oh no, I'll have to go it alone. To ward off mounting apprehension, I spring into action, pretending to be her. I dip the gauze swabs in the bowl of ice water and put them on his eyes.

I give him his pills with some yogurt. He finishes up with apple juice and teddy grahams. He is perky and grateful. By 10 o'clock he is ready to sleep and I put the ointment in his eyes. He is comfortable and prefers to have me sleep next to him in the bed, something I definitely did not want him to do during the first nights of my recovery. It makes it easy for me to get some sleep and still wake up and ice his eyes. He has a good night.

I'm wondering why this is so much easier for him than it was for me. Is it a guy thing?

SATURDAY
Propped up and doped to the gills

Now David feels awful. He can't eat. This has never happened before! Thanks to Sally, I know what to do, and he falls asleep.

I grab the chance to take a shower, and the telephone rings. It's Jaedene. She's calling from her car in my driveway. I dry myself, pull on my shirt and shorts, and go down to say Hi. She sees my red-striped face with no make-up on, the unvarnished truth. (I wouldn't have answered the door to anyone else). She hands me some banana and raspberry baby food. David wakes up, feels better, and eats her comfort food. He takes his next doses without any nausea, then cat-naps through the afternoon.

Kate comes to visit and the sight of him shocks her. She has never seen her Dad slowed down. He never gets sick. Now he is propped up and doped to the gills. Kate sits down beside him and tries to enliven him with ideas she's thinking about. He is trapped. There is no exit for him.

David's mother calls and he can't hear her through the

head bandage. We put her on speakerphone. Right then the children come in to the bedroom arguing and swearing at each other about the mess in the Explorer, the car they both want to use. It is HORRIBLE and they will not stop, nor will they leave the room. I yell at them to get out and I follow them downstairs to talk this out. One refuses to discuss the problem and leaves in the dirty car. The other stays to talk about the situation. I'm jet-lagged, I didn't sleep much, I've been running up and down all day and all night to get ice and food, and I'm exhausted, but I feel sorry that my needs have caused the children inconvenience and pain, and so I sit down and pay attention. At the end of the long conversation I'm devastated to be told I don't listen, can't hear, can't understand, and never get it. I wonder if this ever happens at Jaedene's house? I realize that my children were used to our old faces, that the sight of us is awful, and they feel betrayed, but insight doesn't help. I go back upstairs, sobbing with despair and exhaustion. Taking care of David is much easier than taking care of them — and more appreciated.

SUNDAY
Easier for him
Mercifully I fall asleep early. David has a good night, waking up and going back to sleep, and icing his eyes himself. So, I sleep until I'm wakened at 6 a.m. by loud banging on a bedroom door. The children's fight has recommenced, this time over a radio alarm that should not have gone off. I wish they had meant it when they said that they would never speak to one another again.

By 9:00 a.m. David is sitting up in bed, wearing his glasses at a tilt with a piece of paper towel covering one of the lenses to block his double vision. He is trying to watch television, even though he can't see. His recovery is so much easier than mine was. He likes to say it's because he's the better patient. I think it's because he hasn't had laser treatment. Dr. B says it's because he hasn't had a deep procedure like I had. It's so obvious now that he mentions it.

JAEDENE, MONDAY
The right stuff

I thought I was well into afterwards, and then I noticed Jill's neck didn't look red and feel itchy like mine. My skin doctor said that it was due to injury to the skin around some of the incisions. With the right diagnosis and the right medications, it disappeared in two days.

Then I got an eye irritation and had to go to the ophthalmologist. He said it could be due to a change in the shape of the lid, and the adjustment of the eye to it, like the squeaking of a new wiper on the windshield. With the right diagnosis and the right eye-drops, it disappeared in a day.

JILL, MONDAY
His and hers

It's David's Day 4 and my Day 56. We go to see Dr. B. His and hers appointments! We are in separate rooms and I don't get to see Annie remove David's stitches. When I meet up with him again, his head bandage is off. His eyes are quite purple and his glasses are slanted on his nose. His matted hair is curly and greasy, and he has stubble. He normally NEVER goes out wearing glasses. Today, he looks like a homeless person.

While David is with Annie, Dr. B talks to me alone. He pulls out my pre-surgical photos (how do they get them to look so awful?), compares them to the face before him, and asks me what I think. I agree a lot of my face looks much better, but what about my swollen cheeks? "I'm beginning to think you must have given me implants," I say.

"No, it's all you," he assures me. "It's early yet. The swelling will go down."

He declares that my left eye corner is pulling into shape and he thinks it will make it all the way by itself. If not, in a few months time he'll take a tuck in the eyelid skin, a 30-minute procedure with a 2-day recovery time, but he doesn't think it'll be necessary. He makes it sound like nothing. I wonder.

Dr. B wants to know how my patients are reacting. In particular, since he thinks I look younger (and patients have said the same), he asks how many have come to question my wisdom and my authority. Interesting question, but I haven't noticed any of them wondering about that. Then he wants to know how my family members are taking it.

I tell him, "One child hasn't seen me yet. She comes home tomorrow. The two who are home from college are furious. They think I look like a freak, they wish I hadn't wanted repair, and I feel really bad about it."

"Good," he says. "That means they're idealists. They don't want Mom caring about superficial things like appearance. They want you to be the nurturer. They don't want to see you changing or looking like anything other than over fifty. I think it's fine. I'd rather have kids like that than ones who are trying to please. Your kids are idealistic now, and there's plenty of time for them to change their attitudes about plastic surgery. Eventually your children will have their plastic surgery too, and I guarantee you that they'll be doing it seven years earlier than you did."

TUESDAY
Scary for kids

Xanthe's coming home this morning! "You don't look like Mom," she says. "You look young. I'm supposed to be the young one. Your skin is red and smooth like a baby's. It's weird to leave home with you looking one way and to come back and find you're like a different person. But, even if you're looking younger now it's happening because you are actually getting older, and that means some day you'll die and you won't be here with us. And that's why Zoe and Dan are fighting. We're scared, Mom."

JAEDENE, WEDNESDAY
A guy thing

Now it's Chuck's Day 1. He had his cataract out today. I am all set to take care of him. I ask him how his eye is feeling.

"I can feel it," he says.

What does that mean? I try again. "Does it hurt?"

He just repeats, "I can feel it."

Chuck walks out to the garden and I see him bend down to pick something up, which he's not supposed to do. I knock on the window and say, "No!" He doesn't listen to me. I scream at him, "I'll tell the doctor!" But he feels fine. He was scared of having eye surgery, but now he says it was easy. Jill is going to bring over some baby yogurt for him, but he already wants MEAT.

Chuck doesn't have a Day 1.

He's going to work on Friday and he's going rowing on Saturday. He's going to drive himself to the boat-house. He's talking about his driving, and I'm talking about his denying. The man can't see, and he'll be rowing and driving! Jill says, 'What if he gets a retinal detachment when he's lifting the boat?' I hadn't thought of that. We are all worrying more than he is. He says the doctor says it's okay to row as long as he doesn't hold his breath while pulling or lifting.

I decide to believe him.

Jill, Saturday
Am I naïve, or what?

I'm out with David at lunch with friends. Mandy takes a good look at my face. (No one remarks on David's eyes.) "Jill, your skin looks amazing," she says. "But your cheeks are still swollen. I saw Jaedene at the neighborhood picnic. She doesn't have as much swelling. Keep me posted on how you look when that goes down. I might be thinking of doing something later this year and I might want your surgeon's name. My mother's skin was beautiful to the day she died, but mine is more like my father's. My Daddy's skin had fallen down past his chin, and that's why I might need to do something."

"Same in my family," I say.

"When he died, the funeral home padded his cheeks to take up the skin. Weird."

I feel horribly self-conscious about my swollen cheeks. I hope she doesn't think I've been embalmed.

"So I think I'll need to get my neck done," she goes on.

Remembering what Jaedene told me, I say, "You did your eyes before, didn't you? They look good." (And they do.)

"No, I didn't. I've never had anything done," she says. "It's Jaedene who had her eyes done before. Not that she told me, but that was the scuttlebutt around the neighborhood."

That's the same thing Jaedene said about her! Now I really begin to wonder what I'm getting into. Is it that Mandy is dissembling or that Jaedene isn't telling me everything? Are they in the know or just being catty? Or am I naïve? The only answer I can be sure of is that I'm naïve.

I ask Jaedene about it and she's upset that I doubted her.

A Small Care Package for a Friend

- *Children's toothbrush and toothpaste*
- *Johnson's no-tears shampoo and detangler*
- *Crabtree and Evelyn face blotting paper*
- *Vaseline lip-balm*
- *A packet of teddy graham crackers*
- *People magazine*
- *Video of My Fair Lady*
- *A CD of her/his favorite music*

Jaedene, Saturday
Ruth's Day 4

Eight weeks after my surgery, Ruth had a facelift. She's the friend who sent me the care package. Then I sent her a care package, and now I'm sending her ME. I go visit Ruth to give her another kind of lift — emotional as well as visual. I figure that seeing me, she will know that in eight weeks or so she too will be fine.

But Ruth is already "fine!" She just doesn't know it. True, she is swollen, and the lasered area above her lip is red, but she is definitely ten days ahead of where I was at only four days post-op. Because she had her eyes done five years ago, she had only a small "tuck" taken on her upper lids on this go-round. Her surgery lasted for two hours, while mine took eight. The sides of her face are packed in ice, and I was never packed in anything other than bandages on the first night. Her incisions differ from mine also. She has skin gathered behind her earlobe, with the incision coming down in front of the ear and below the lobe, and nothing in the hairline anywhere. She has not had a browlift. And she had no laser below her eyes. Even the laser doesn't look too bad — relatively speaking. She sits at her dining room table with me and EATS A LOT of REAL FOOD, in fact, chunky chicken and everything else I eat for lunch.

Ruth is taking three homeopathic medications, and I had only taken Arnica. She has a specially formulated treatment cream with retin-A and glycolic acid that the pharmacist has to make up. This she must use after washing her face, and before putting on her special moisturizer. The pharmacist is not happy about this special cream. He says it is a pain to concoct, and Jill says she'd rather have surgery than that stuff on her face.

Ruth's day nurse — who by the way looks terrific eight weeks after her own facelift — took care of a middle-Eastern QUEEN, after HER facelift. I am starting to feel like the proverbial "country cousin." But, that's okay, because Ruth is happy and relieved to see me, and I feel the same about her.

I tell Chuck that Ruth looks great. What I mean is, she doesn't look like she has been in a war the way Jill and I did. Chuck tells me again how horrible I looked and how scared he was. I feel sad. I feel sorry for him. He had to look at me even when I couldn't.

Connecting Through a Facelift

There's nothing like caring for your husband or your friend to take your mind off your own troubles. Seeing a man deal with fear in "guy fashion" is a bit annoying. Remind yourself, he wouldn't have it so easy if he had to contend with a full facelift. Helping your friend brings satisfaction and also feelings of competition. Helping gives you one of the things you were hoping for – connection.

14

There and Getting There

Month 4 for us,
Days 5 and 19 for Chuck and David

*W*E HAVE A DATE WITH OUR HUSBANDS FOR DINNER. CHUCK IS NOT THE LEAST BOTHERED by the fact that his eye is bloodshot. If you ask him if it hurts, he doesn't know. David has been teaching workshops in Korea, paying no attention to the fact that his eyes still have purple rims and are slanted, but then getting a kick out of his Korean hosts finding his eyes more attractive than in his advance publicity photograph.

David and Chuck like to joke about us. Chuck calls Jaedene his trophy wife and David says he's getting a new wife without having to go through another divorce. They don't seem to need our sympathy. They are thinking more about being with us than how we feel being out with them.

On Chuck's Day 2 he was back at work. On Day 3, he was already rowing. On David's Day 4 he was out for a walk, and on Day 7 he went back to work a week early. On his Day 21, David flew to Korea to teach for the weekend. On his Day 16, Chuck was competing with 7200 rowers in Montreal.

It's not that the men are braver than we are. It's just that they didn't have what we had and they don't care how they look. No, they do like to look attractive, but if they don't for any reason, it doesn't bother them. They're male, no matter what, and that's enough for them to feel secure.

*j*ILL
Ruth's rapid refill

Hearing about Ruth's speedy recovery, I can see why some people ask for the New York lift. Dr. B says it has to be done again in three to five years. Ruth's already doing the next step. She's going for Botox injections to soften the wrinkling of her forehead and collagen injections to fill in below her eyes. Jaedene and I preferred to get it all over with at one time. But we may have to go in for some fine tuning too before our surgeons are satisfied.

It's nice to have the choice of a short-term surface-lift or a long-term deep-tissue lift. A television star could never have the kind of facelift I've had or she would be off the screen for at least three months.

What about me?

It's been more than three months, but it's still not afterwards for me yet. I still have one scab above my ear. My face no longer twangs and twizzles, but my scalp still itches. I no longer have the false impression I need to brush hair away from my left eye. My laser streaks are fading but still need to be covered with foundation. My regular one will do. I am still swollen, but my teeth look like my own again, and I no longer look like a freak.

My step-daughter Nell comes down from New York and sees me for the first time. She is impressed. "You look so young," she says.

This is not what I had bargained for. Rested and refreshed is what Jaedene and I were aiming at. In the elevator at the doctor's office a man I'd call young, in his thirties, actually struck up a conversation with me. When I told Jaedene, she said she had become visible too. Do they see us because of how we look? Or have we been making ourselves invisible because of how we felt we looked? Whatever the reason, I tell Nell that being seen as younger is quite something to get used to.

Looking younger and getting attention from men is something we've noticed and we get a kick out of it. Nell wants us to look the way we want, but as a younger woman she wishes we didn't care. She wants us to get more out of our facelifts than male attention. Didn't we find wisdom and insight? Yes, we found a great deal to reflect on. Didn't we feel sad that our culture doesn't show more respect for age and wisdom and doesn't find beauty in aging? Yes, it's sad. But at least our culture allows me to be a physician and have a facelift if I please.

jAEDENE
Guilty?

Jill and I have been looking at each other, talking with each other, supporting each other, and writing together for more than three months. But we have not healed at the same rate. There is too much contrast in how each of us looks at this point. This has been difficult for both of us. I feel concerned for Jill. I want her to be farther along in the process, so she can enjoy the benefits of what she has chosen to do. Our results and our experiences right now aren't comparable.

I want us to be able to enjoy the benefits TOGETHER. I feel as though I have gone on without her to a certain extent. I didn't sign up to do that, and I feel guilty about it. Jill has referred to it as "Facelift Survivor's Guilt." But I don't think that truly fits, because she WILL catch up. So, I have decided to name it "Quicker-Healing Guilt" — and blame it on the doctors.

jILL
Race you to the finish

Jaedene recovered much faster than I did, and Ruth is going to recover faster than Jaedene. It doesn't seem fair. But Jaedene and I both had an in-depth approach and that is supposed to last longer. That had better be true. We want Ruth to be happy, but, after the hours of surgery we've been through, we want to know there is SOME difference.

I asked Dr. B why I was taking so long to heal. He reminded me that he had said some faces take six months to a year. Yes, he had said that. Everything he said was borne out in my experience. I guess I just didn't take it in because it had no emotional impact. (That's why we think you need a book like this.) Dr. B said, "Recovery from the complete facelift at the deepest level is hard work." I like that. I can stop thinking of myself as a complainer and think of myself as a hard worker!

Jaedene and I wanted to go through this together but we're feeling separated by our different rates of healing now. Talking together is great but comparing our progress is not. We each had good surgeons who gave us in-depth approaches at the level each of us chose, but the difference in our outcomes is a strain on both of us. One way of being together is to unite in claiming our right to a better result than Ruth should expect. But I was on the table one hour longer than Jaedene and I'm taking much longer to recover a normal face. By that argument, I deserve a better result than Jaedene. She feels guilty about acknowledging the difference in improvement between us, and I feel guilty about secretly wishing I were the one who is guilty about looking better.

15

Back on the Table

jILL, MONTH 5
It's nothing?

DR. B EXAMINES ME INTENTLY. "IT LOOKS GOOD," HE SAYS. I SMILE. He continues, "So now it's time for a little fine tuning." My face falls. "You'll just have to trust me. No cost to you. This is what completes the job — add a little fat below the eyes, remove some extra skin on the upper eye-lids and scar tissue behind the ear-lobes. We'll do it in the office, under local, takes half an hour, a two-day recovery. It's nothing." I make the appointment for a Thursday to give me two days to be ready for my Saturday night out.

When the day comes, I'm remembering Jaedene's friend who said that her "nothing" procedure had hurt like hell! Annie gives me some Valium and Xanax. She begins with lidocaine injections to freeze my hip for taking the fat to put in my face. Indeed that's nothing. Then she injects lidocaine into my face. "This'll burn and sting," she says. I know that. I can handle that. That's nothing. But it just keeps on going, one injection after another. Suddenly I just crumple and cry, "I can't take this." I feel humiliated, defeated, and ashamed of myself. Hadn't I had three children without any anesthetic? Didn't my dentist tell me I have a high pain threshold? Crying is not how I think of myself at all. Annie says it happens all the time, probably because of the medication. Dr. B says, "We can leave the rest for another time ..." I say, "No! Whatever you're doing, do it now — because I'm never coming back." He gives me some more Valium, and I don't remember any more until it's all over.

When I get home I sleep for three hours, and when I waken I can't remember anything about the drive home or the pretty carnations Jaedene sent. I feel fine but the next morning I take a nose-dive. I can't keep anything down. The bandage feels hot and uncomfortable — the dreaded bathing-cap-chin-strap feeling is back, and I have a relentlessly miserable day. Next day I'm fine and I get to take off the bandage. I look like I've stepped four months back. I have swollen, bruised eyes with black stitches, a bruised mouth, and pinhole scars on my cheeks and chin. I'm going out Saturday night anyway because I'll be sitting in the dark at a movie, but I better look a whole lot better by Tuesday when I go back to work. I don't want to re-traumatize my patients.

Tuesday comes and I'm still bruised, scabby, and swollen. A dear colleague has died and the reception is tonight. I'm not allowed to wear make-up and I look awful, but I don't want to miss it. When one of the guests tells me I shouldn't be kissing people because I have "open wounds that could be infected," I feel disgusting, and crawl home.

jILL, MONTH 6
Disconcerting but not so bad

David is glad my eyes look more like mine again. My left cheek is closer to normal size, but my scalp is still itching, my nose is too wide, my left eye still has a wrinkle that wasn't there before, like a stitch is pulling, and my upper lip is slightly swollen.

Six weeks later, I decide I probably look better to others than I think, and I decide to give a party for my women friends. Jaedene is here, and so is her friend Ruth. They both look like themselves, only better, and I can't figure out how. No-one at the party can tell that they had anything done. Jaedene had told her doctor that she wanted to be able to complain that he hadn't done enough. Ruth had told her doctor that she should look like she hadn't gotten her money's worth. They both got exactly what they wanted.

I hadn't wanted anything so precise. Basically I just asked Dr. B to do whatever needed doing. I got more than I bargained for. Sitting next to me, Judy says, "Jill, you look terrific, but it's disconcerting. I have to remind myself it's you." That really sums it up.

At a conference, students were surprised by my appearance. One told me that I now looked really great, but another said she was angry at losing the face that was familiar. A woman was crying because she used to feel close to me on account of the fact that she saw a similarity between her mother and me, and now she could no longer find her mother's face in my face. Having the facelift made me realize how the students are attached to me as a mother figure, and how much comfort they had found in the signs of aging that let me fit the mold. To many people my face is disconcerting.

This does embarrass me, but it's getting to be a bit of a kick, at least around here.

Now Scotland is another matter. I'm going there next week for my mother's birthday. I've tried to warn her I look different, but she pretends that no one will notice. I wonder if she'll miss the face she has known longer than anyone else. I'm glad she thinks I look "not too bad at all." My friend Jenny stands me in front of the long mirror on top of the fireplace. She looks carefully at me in the glass as I look at her. She's almost my age, but her chin and neck are fine. Her face, however, is swollen as a result of medication she has to take because of a serious medical problem. We both express regret that the other's face doesn't look the way we remembered. She's a generous person and she concludes that my facelift is brilliant.

MONTH 7
It's nothing, #2

David has been great. When I've complained, 'My face still looks swollen,' he's been saying, 'I'm so pleased you had it done. You look so much better.' Today when I say, "It's much less saggy, but what bothers me is that my face looks fake," he finally admits, "You're right. It doesn't look quite natural, but I can't figure out what it is that causes that." It's a relief to know that I didn't imagine it, but now what do I do?

I see Dr. B for my check-up. "Your nostrils have had some lateral excursion, so I need to pull them in a little," he says, "and I still need to get another millimetre of lift on the left eye-brow. It's still too low. I don't know why I didn't get it last time, but it needs doing. We'll get you on the schedule for two months from now. It's nothing." I've heard that before, and I guess I'm getting used to it, because I just accept the news this time. But I notice I don't exactly run to make an appointment.

MONTH 9
Final nip and tuck

I go in for what I hope will be my final nip and tuck. I trust I won't emerge looking even less natural. Working under local as before, Dr. B trims the excess above my eyelid, smoothes out the wrinkle to the left of my left eye, and pulls in my nostrils. Annie holds the Xanax, and with only Valium and Hydrocodone on board, I stay awake the whole time, all the better to tell you what is happening. The injections on the temple do sting and burn, but those on the eyelids are nothing at all. Then the nose. Omigod, the nose! 4 shots to numbing, and I nearly jump off the table. Then I feel cutting and stitching that pulls like a drawstring, but no more pain. At one point, Dr. B asks Annie to pass the screwdriver. SCREWDRIVER! Yes, the little screws are still in there and he's going to tighten them and so pull my tissues into place as if on a winch. Annie tells me that some women go in there and act like it's no big deal. Lucky for them.

Back home, I ice assiduously day and night for 24 hours and manage to avoid swelling. I am bruised around the eyes but the rest of me looks fine. I have a much easier recovery this time, but I can't watch television for long or read small print. Jaedene is out of town giving a paper, so I can't call her. I feel bored and sleepy. David is bored too, but he wants to keep me company, so he is watching the basketball game on our bedroom television. I am ready to kill him.

Monday, I go back to work only slightly bruised and I feel fine.

MONTH 11

All of a sudden, my healing is complete. At her graduation, my daughter tells me I look beautiful. I am glad for that, but I still feel that I look fake.

MONTH 14

Over the summer my face continues settling. To my enormous relief, I stop looking fake. I don't feel self-conscious any more. Friends no longer comment on my appearance. My mother says I look like her daughter. I look like myself. I'm there at last!

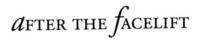

*a*FTER THE *f*ACELIFT

16

Final Word of Wisdom

Why the aging face may need a facelift

*W*HEN WE WERE YOUNG WE WERE SURE THAT THERE WAS SOMETHING QUITE WONDERFUL about seeing life experience etched in the lines of the face. As we got older we agreed that some people age beautifully but we found that we were not among them. Our faces were sending the wrong messages about us. When Jill was concentrating or puzzled, her frown made her seem angry or disapproving. Jaedene's low eyebrows made her look tired. Mouth corners that turned down gave us a grumpy look. Due to the hormonal changes of aging, we lost fat around the eyes, in the upper cheeks, and in the lips, and it fell into wrinkles around the mouth, chin, and neck. We looked less feminine. The extra skin and fat got in the way of the proper relationship between eyes, nose, and mouth. Our eyes seemed smaller and the feelings that they expressed were less obvious. It was harder for people to read us when our eyes, the windows of the soul, were half-closed. Unhappy with the way our faces were aging, we looked worse. It was a vicious cycle.

The effect of our choice on our children

Watching a mother recover from a facelift is too gross for comfort for children, even ones who are grown, especially daughters. Choosing a facelift makes them worry that we don't feel as attractive as they think we should. Worse than that, it reminds them of our age, and our eventual death. There is nothing harder for a child to bear. Zoe said that she kept thinking of James Joyce's phrase "One life. One body. Do. But do" to which she wanted to add, "But don't do THIS!" They were frightened of the procedure. As Zoe said, "Blood and guts should be, and stay, on the inside."

They may take some pleasure from watching parents take care of one another, but children feel excluded and inadequate. Even adult children are terrified by the physical signs and emotional vulnerability of the healing process. They realize that we are in no position to take care of them, and it's hard for them to look at us, much less take care of us and accept our choices. Even if they do not come home until after recovery, when they do, they may have to deal with the shock of a parent with an unfamiliar face. Zoe, who lived through the recovery process, would have preferred to watch Jill age gently, and keep her familiar face, than to have her change drastically. On a positive note, however, Stephanie, who came home after healing was complete, found Jaedene's reconstructed face more recognizable than before because it was similar to the one she had lived with on a daily basis, which was at least fifteen years ago.

Zoe and Stephanie swear up and down that they will never subject themselves to the indignity of a facelift, but as Zoe acknowledges, "I guess society, and my mother, would put five dollars on the other side of that bet."

What the facelift can do

Some women with wrinkles feel beautiful and they remain attractive. But in our society, age is not given respect, and there is a double standard by which women are judged more harshly than men. Since we are affected by our social groups and our culture, many of us feel the need to enhance what nature gave and to hide what age brings. Make-up helps us look the way we want. Smiling helps to lift the face naturally, but we can't always be smiling. As we get older, make-up can't accomplish what it used to do for us. That's where cosmetic surgery comes in.

A facelift can't turn the clock back, but it interrupts the cycle of frowning and worrying about it. A facelift can't reverse menopause but it can counteract the effect of changing hormone levels on the facial contours. A facelift can't make you happy if you aren't and it can't make you into a beauty, but it can erase some of the signs of aging that get in the way of looking as vital, feminine, and attractive as you feel.

The face that fits "the inner me"

The male face ages too, but society doesn't care about that. No matter how old a man is, he is still a man and he doesn't have to worry about being unattractive. Female faces in our society suffer from the signs of aging more than male faces, and then women feel less attractive and less feminine.

We women usually live longer — so our faces have more time to show signs of age. By the time we're in our fifties, we notice these changes — if we haven't already seen them coming in our forties.

Not all of us lose our looks, but many do. Not all of us wish away the signs of age, but many do. Some of us who feel that looking older makes us unattractive fear that we will be left. A facelift won't prevent that if it's going to happen, but it makes us feel more attractive and less disenfranchised. Feeling good about our appearance helps us to enjoy getting older. It's worth it to invest in ourselves, and having a facelift is another way of doing that. A facelift can't ever make us young, or even look as if we are young again, but it can restore features that are lost as we age. Some women even claim that it helps them keep their jobs!

We each wanted a facelift to give us back the external face to match the inner person. We wanted to maintain our self-confidence in our appearance, our desirability to our partners, our marketability in the work-place, and our visibility in the worlds of work and social life.

Dealing with compliments and flattery

A compliment seems like a dangerous indicator of what might possibly happen. If we appear more desirable, others in our presence might feel less so, and therefore, we could possibly be rejected. Also, if we believe the compliment, could we somehow come to rely too much on how we look, and not enough on what we think and do? It takes time to learn how to accept compliments if they haven't been coming our way for a while. And we know, after watching our faces age to date, and particularly as they inevitably continue to do so after our surgery, that the lines will reappear. We will continue to age, but we hope that our facelifts will allow us to do so more gracefully.

Being your best

There are many kinds of female power — professional, social, sexual, and parental. With power you can make things happen. There's a lot to be said for it, and beauty is one way to get it. Those of us who are not great beauties need to work on looking our best. Being attractive brings opportunities, connections, and satisfaction to men and women. The more attractive a woman is, the more attention she gets, more privileges become available, more opportunities, and therefore, more choices. But beauty alone won't suffice. Beauty is only skin deep. You have to have what it takes to build on the initial attractiveness. If you work on who you are, you want a face to match. That's why you have a facelift.

What you see in the facelift mirror

Having a facelift pulls you into a journey of self-discovery and self-revelation. It makes you think about your face and what it means to you and others. Your face marks your identity. The physical transformation of your face affects the way you experience yourself and the way other people see you. Outer improvement brings inner transformation. That's why you have it done.

17

What About You?

ONCE YOU GET THE THOUGHT IN YOUR HEAD THAT YOUR FACE NEEDS HELP, THE THOUGHT STAYS THERE. You don't look at yourself the next morning and say, "You know, I look fine."

How can you afford it?

High costs are an issue for many women. Not everyone can afford it. A facelift used to be only for the rich and famous. That was long ago. Now people like us can do this. If it's important to you, you make it a priority. You can always work out a monthly payment plan, or you can put the charges on a credit card. That's the American way. You can have what you want and then pay it off over time. The other thing is that the price is not as high outside a big city and outside the United States, for instance in South America.

What if you are a man?

A man doesn't need a facelift to be recognized. The pressure isn't on you in the same way. You have facial hair, and you can cover your face in ways that a woman cannot. But if your eyes are encroached on by lids drooping above, and bags below, or eyes bulging in shrinking sockets, you might want to have an eyelift. If the skin above your collar is loose, you might want to have it neatened. Many older men with young children have mentioned to us that they wish to have their necks done to look younger. On the other hand, a man looking younger might look less powerful, and that's a reason you might not want it. Women like men to look older. Look at the wrinkles on the Marlborough Man. Last word, a man is a man, and that's often enough!

Finding the kind of facelift you want

There are various facelifts -- long, short, surface, deep, pulled up or out, scars in front, in, or behind the ear, part or all of the face and neck -- and many different techniques to carry them out. You can find the one that is appropriate for you

---

Choosing your facelift

Let's say you choose to proceed with having a facelift. Depending on the look you want to achieve, you need to decide whether to ask for a conservative restoration or a radical improvement, a surface lift or a deep-tissue lift, a traditional incision or a modified short-scar facelift. What you choose is determined by your age, how much time you can afford to give your recovery, and the look you want to achieve. You may decide on a strategy of repeat procedures, a little at a time, or do the whole thing just once. The more thorough your procedure the longer your recovery takes.

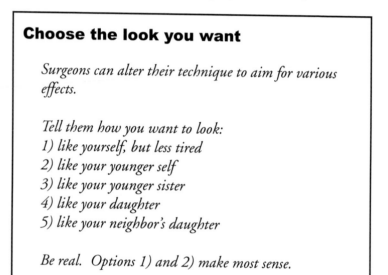

Choose the look you want

Surgeons can alter their technique to aim for various effects.

Tell them how you want to look:
1) like yourself, but less tired
2) like your younger self
3) like your younger sister
4) like your daughter
5) like your neighbor's daughter

Be real. Options 1) and 2) make most sense.

Healing

You will notice that while you are healing, from day to day you have a different experience of yourself, and people respond in various ways. Some may feel scared looking at your still-in-process face, especially those who are thinking of a lift themselves. If they don't want a lift, they wonder if you are counting their wrinkles. Most of all they just don't know what to make of your appearance. You have gone from being as familiar as an old shoe to being an unknown quantity, momentarily looking worse, frightening, or even alien.

It's disconcerting to look at yourself in the mirror. Other people notice that your face isn't quite right. You look lop-sided, because each side of the face heals at a different rate. A symmetrical face is considered beautiful, especially when there is a subtle irregularity to emphasize its basic integrity. But your asymmetry isn't subtle and that's why your expressions may look forced, slightly "off," perhaps even ugly.

While you are healing you may look like, and feel like, someone you are not, because your improving face gives a false advertisement about who you are. If you look awful, you may feel you should hide, even if you don't really want to. If you look great, some people may feel that you have gained an unfair advantage, and you, yourself, may worry that your concern for looking good may hurt them. Friends and associates may start thinking of you as shallow, weak, and vain. If you can change so easily, perhaps you're not to be trusted. They may wonder if you will change again, or change your feelings as well as your face, and decide to leave them behind, as surely as you've turned your back on your old face.

If your new appearance doesn't fit with your inner sense of yourself, you are in for a confusing time. If it does fit with how you feel but not with how you think others feel about you, you may feel disoriented, scared, or depressed. If you look a whole lot better or younger, you may feel elated. Whatever form they take, your feelings will be intense and fluctuating. Talk about them with a friend, and if that doesn't work, find a psychotherapist with a good understanding of plastic surgery.

Anxiously watching your healing take place, you may worry that you are so preoccupied with your looks that you will lose touch with the deeper aspects of your self. The inner self needs as much attention as the face. Healing the body and taking care of your inner self take time — and we mean months, not weeks.

What about your children?

When their own identity is still forming or in transition during a crisis, children find a slightly unfamiliar parent especially disconcerting. They may not be able to take care of you, or even to look at you. Try to understand their aversion not as a rejection, but as a token of respect and love. Let them help at a distance, by finding you CDs, getting books on tape from the local library, and searching for your favorite flavor of baby food. What's best for them is to be out of the house, preferably at a good place in their lives. Here is Jaedene's daughter Stephanie's advice:

Do not get a face-lift at the following times:

1) During a child's freshman year in college
2) During a child's pregnancy
3) During a child's divorce

Your children want to know that you have considered the impact on them. It's even better if you can protect them from seeing you too soon. Even if they have to be at home, they benefit from seeing how you make choices and take care of yourself inside and out, and from how you accept the support of your husband, partner, or friends.

Matching inner and outer self

A facelift lets you match your face to your view of yourself. If your inner self is in good shape, a wonderful feeling of harmony and confidence follows. This is the best reason to have a facelift.

How long will your facelift last?

How long your facelift will last depends on many factors — which lift you had done, how tight your surgeon pulled, and your age. A deep lift lasts longer than a surface lift — some say 10-15 years instead of 5-7 years. If you are over sixty, you age and sag faster than if you are younger at the time of the operation. No facelift lasts forever, and you will continue to age afterwards. The result will not be perfect. You will be happier with it if you already feel good about yourself and enjoy your life. A facelift does not transform reality, but it certainly can enhance it. It's good to be realistic, and then you'll be satisfied.

What's the impact on your emotions and your identity?

Let's say you, like Jill, have more or less healed at two months and you're ready to see people, but you still don't look like yourself. Some people may feel comfortable with you, but others may feel fear, pity or contempt for how you look. Some may be threatened by how great they imagine you are going to look. Your children who feel a sense of ownership of your face may feel robbed. Some of Jill's patients (who have the privilege of saying what social friends can't) reported feeling that she had become like a stranger. Like those patients and those children, some of the people who know you well may not feel as intimate with you as they did before you became this stranger who does whatever she wants.

Or if you, like Jaedene, have healed nicely and your appearance is improved at two months, people who don't know you will treat you in new ways. Doors may open. Let's say your face looks younger than before surgery: People will judge you as more energetic and more able than when you had the older face. Let's say you look more attractive: You'll be dealing with desire and therefore envy. You'll receive compliments and favorable treatment, just as cute babies get more hugs, attractive children get better grades, and good-looking women employees command higher salaries. If your new look matches your mental outlook, you feel secure in this recognition.

Reflecting on your experience

It takes looking at all of your reflections to understand why having a facelift is a big deal. It may even feel like too much at times. The facelift involves the past, present, and future. It reverberates with every aspect of life as a woman, a wife, a daughter, and a mother (and with the equivalent roles for a man). The facelift is a test of fortitude and a challenge to identity. You have feelings of uncertainty, anxious anticipation, and some depression. That's why it is so helpful to go through it with a friend. That's why we are sharing our experiences.

As you and your friend learn more about the face, the facelift, the process of recovery, and how each of you feels, your relationship deepens and you come to understand more about yourselves. As your face settles and you get used to the form it now has, you explore new experiences of yourself in all your relationships. You have a new outlook on the world. You enjoy your face and the insight it brings you.

We hope that our diaries will encourage you to join us on this journey of self-discovery as we all follow face and fortune into the future.

18

Beginning: The New Face

JAEDENE
Yes, I'm glad I did it

THREE WEEKS AFTER THE SURGERY, CHUCK AND I VISITED FRIENDS IN NEW YORK WHERE OUR DAUGHTERS LIVE. Our younger daughter Stephanie came to see me. She was immediately relieved to see that I still look like myself. However, she didn't want to know any details of the surgery, and she didn't want to look at where the incisions were around my face or in my scalp. Our older daughter Marjorie was away on vacation and so she didn't see me, and she didn't ask about the facelift. My husband was still thinking I was crazy for doing it, but that I looked great.

Six weeks afterwards, when I visited my mother, she said again that I didn't need it. She wasn't curious about what or how it was done. My great aunt was fascinated and thrilled for me. She moved a lamp near my face, and studied it, wanting to know every detail.

At eight weeks, I went back to New York. Marjorie finally saw my face. She said she was very relieved and happy that I looked like myself, and that I looked good. She pointed out a new dimple in my chin, and said she liked it. I didn't know it was there. We were sitting in a restaurant together, talking about my face and catching up on all her news. A couple was sitting at the table behind us, but we barely noticed them. I went to the ladies room, and, while I was gone, they started talking to her. When I returned, she introduced us. The couple could not believe she was sitting with her MOTHER.

Part of the reason was that I didn't look old, but the other was that my daughter and I had been engrossed in conversation for so long it seemed that we were friends. They didn't have those times with their mothers, they explained. That part made me feel sad for them and very happy for me.

On the train returning to Washington, two younger men introduced themselves at different times, making efforts to start and continue conversations. I had to stop myself from saying, "Don't you realize that I'm much too old for you?"

At three months, walking home after dinner with Chuck one evening, I was amazed when two men stopped to look at me, said I looked gorgeous, and told Chuck to hold on to me. There's something to be said for a facelift ...

At four months, my husband was calling me his trophy wife.

At five months, my husband is still calling me his trophy wife, as in beautiful and MUCH younger.

There's a lot to be said for a facelift.

JILL
Lady in waiting

At one week, I was tired and my face looked burned and alien.

At two weeks, I got energetic and exhausted myself. I covered the burns with make-up, but my face looked android.

At three weeks, I had energy to see friends but I found it hard to do. I could put in my lenses and use make-up. My cheeks were swollen like an eggplant colored red.

At weeks four and five, my face was still distorted. I went out but I felt uncomfortable in sun or heat.

At six weeks, I was traveling, and meeting people. I was looking greasy and feeling socially uncomfortable. I was working hard emotionally and being extremely self-protective.

At seven weeks, I wanted to be finished like Jaedene, but I was not. I was feeling depressed and envious.

At two months I was back at work, looking younger but swollen. Some patients felt that they were talking to a stranger. I kept wishing I looked like myself. I thought, "This is hard work."

At three months I was getting compliments, but my face was still slightly swollen and shiny. There was a scab above one ear. My hair was still a mess. I needed a make-up artist to help me adjust to my new face.

At four months, I looked more like myself again, but I was still a bit swollen. My hair was better, but still weak. My scalp itched, but cortisone mousse helped. I didn't yet look the way I wanted to, but I could see that I would. I was feeling more relaxed. Having patience was the hardest work of all.

At five months, I looked much better and got a new haircut. A playwright cast me as Mussolini's blonde mistress for his play-reading the next season. My former analyst said I looked great, and surprised me by revealing that she used to imagine having a facelift.

At six months, I had some fine-tuning. It helped but it didn't get me all the way. I looked good, but I looked fake.

At eight months, I had my second nip and tuck. I looked more like me.

At 14 months my face finally settled in. My mother said I look like her daughter again. I read the role of Mussolini's mistress. Now I'm having fun!

The last word

It's not that we look much younger than we did before the facelift, it's that we don't look so marked by age. And, because we don't, we don't look the same, period. There is no middle: If my face has changed, I have changed. Having a facelift, we cross a line, and we can't go back. But that doesn't mean that we are dismissing friends who don't want a facelift. We can connect, and we still want to, and we still want them. But we're glad we look tons better and that gives us confidence for facing the future. A facelift is a new beginning.

JAEDENE

Parts of my face, scalp and neck will be numb
For a LONG time
My face looks most different
When I'm not in a setting I'm used to
I'm glad when people don't know about my facelift
On the other hand, I'm disappointed
And I want to tell them
I'm looking at younger looking clothes
I am just beginning to comprehend that I am changed
 FOREVER
There's envy to deal with
    Back-handed compliments
    Whispers and nudges
I feel confused when people look at me
I wonder if they are studying my facelift
I wonder if they can see ME
My friends are generally supportive
They tell me what they need to do to their faces
Then they say they probably never will ...
Yeah. Right.
Knowing what I know now, would I have second thoughts?
Yes, I would have second thoughts
And then I would have it done.